Doctor Morrison's
Miracle Body Tune-Up
for Rejuvenated Health

Doctor Morrison's
Miracle Body Tune-Up
for Rejuvenated Health

Marsh Morrison, D.C., Ph.C., F.I.C.C.

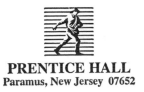

PRENTICE HALL
Paramus, New Jersey 07652

Library of Congress Cataloging-in-Publication Data

Morrison, Marsh.
    Doctor Morrison's miracle body tune-up for
rejuvenated health.
      ISBN 0-13-216366-7
      1. Hygiene.   2. Exercise—Physiological
effect.   3. Massage.   I. Title.
    [DNLM: 1. Medicine—Popular works.   WB120 M881d
1973]
RA776.5.M63   1973   73-7976
613.7′1   CIP

Printed in the United States of America

40 39 38 37 36 35 34 33 32

This book is a reference work based on research by the author. The opinions expressed herein are not necessarily those of or endorsed by the publisher. The directions stated in this book are in no way to be considered as a substitute for consultation with a duly licensed doctor.

ISBN 0-13-216366-7

ATTENTION: CORPORATIONS AND SCHOOLS

Prentice Hall books are available at quantity discounts with bulk purchase for educational, business, or sales promotional use. For information, please write to: Prentice Hall Career & Personal Development Special Sales, 240 Frisch Court, Paramus, New Jersey 07652. Please supply: title of book, ISBN number, quantity, how the book will be used, date needed.

PRENTICE HALL
Career & Personal Development
Paramus, NJ 07652
A Simon & Schuster Company

On the World Wide Web at http://www.phdirect.com

Prentice-Hall International (UK) Limited, *London*
Prentice-Hall of Australia Pty. Limited, *Sydney*
Prentice-Hall Canada Inc., *Toronto*
Prentice-Hall Hispanoamericana, S.A., *Mexico*
Prentice-Hall of India Private Limited, *New Delhi*
Prentice-Hall of Japan, Inc., *Tokyo*
Simon & Schuster Asia Pte. Ltd., *Singapore*
Editora Prentice-Hall do Brasil, Ltda., *Rio de Janeiro*

Other books by Dr. Marsh Morrison:

They Called Him Doctor
City of Fingerless Men
If I Were a Chiropractor's Wife
The Climate of Passion
The Impossible Doctor Butch

Dr. Morrison is also the author of a scientific scmimonthly newsletter, "The Marsh Morrison International Report," for professional use.

This Book Is Dedicated

To the sick who are sick of being sick,

And to the lost and frightened ones who are still sick after sampling the conventional hospitals, drugs and doctors,

And to those who do not know where to turn now that drugs and surgeries have failed them, believing wrongly that medical doctoring is the only kind of doctoring that exists,

And to those who see their cuts and bruises healing without the aid of doctors and know that the body is a self-healing organism, and because "the heart knows reasons that reason cannot understand" they have hope for a *natural* kind of health that is not what Alexis Carrel called "the nonlasting *artificial* health that depends upon hospitals, drugs and doctors,"

To all these I dedicate this book . . . because it is a volume that opens the door to at least some measure of health for all, containing the time-tested results of over forty years of disciplined original researches.

M. M.

What This Book
Can Do For You

Are you sick of being sick? Many people are. I have talked to them during a 35-city lecture tour of the United States and Canada, and know what they think. They are disgusted. It costs so very much to get well. And then, usually, they don't even *get* well. We know there's a lot of fanfare about the *imminent* cure of this-and-that disease. But the fact is that health disorder is the order of the day.

What's wrong? There must be something missing. The doctors know a lot of things, that is certain. But are they *doing* the right things? If they are, then why do we have this continually rising incidence of heart disease, cancer, mental illness, muscular dystrophy, multiple sclerosis, epilepsy, cerebral palsy, diabetes, arthritis, cystic fibrosis, Parkinson's disease, kidney disease, and so on? It must stand to reason that our doctors are *missing* something; they must be failing to do what the sick people need to have done for them.

If you cut your skin or break a bone the body heals itself. The human system tends toward the normal; it *wants* to be well. So if we ever got hold of the *Missing Health Link* in doctoring, this "something extra" that's needed by men and women who are sick, then we could expect less heart disease and mental illness and cancer and all the rest.

The fact is that there is *A Missing Health Link.* At last we have found it and know what it is. We know what the doctors have been missing—what they've been failing to do for the sick, the lost and frightened, and helpless.

"Nature cures and the doctor pockets the fee," said Ben Franklin. In the light of present physiological knowledge it appears that people tend to get well by themselves. It is the nature of the body to heal itself, and we doctors have been getting the credit for cures which we did not bring about.

The great news is that *The Missing Health Link* that I speak about can in most cases be applied by *you* to yourself. Only in very rare instances will you need the services of a doctor, if you read and follow this Missing Health Link program. Even then, should there be a dire emergency or grave illness and you need the aid of a doctor, the fact that you knew the Missing Link program and applied it to yourself will make the doctor's efforts in your behalf so much easier.

So I have written this book for *you,* and with a full, hopeful heart and mind I urge you to *read* it and *heed* it. It is for *you*; and it is for all those you care about. When you—or they—are sick (and nearly all of us get sick in *some* way in these upside-down times), you will find in the pages of this book some very straight answers: all the things about getting well that you've always wanted to know about and never expected to get your hands on.

My patients ask me, "What *exactly* can I do for my health, Dr. Morrison? I am constipated. I always get sore throats, I have asthma, I'm hard of hearing. Or it's an embarrassing skin rash, or headaches from eyestrain, or I've got a chronic appendicitis or a spinal disc problem. Any answers?"

My answer is a confident, "Yes." This book is full of answers to these and other health problems, both common and uncommon. Those mentioned above, for example: the way the research scholar from Formosa conquered his *constipation* by the use of ordinary apples and the pectin therein (chapter 6); or the way one pronounces the vowels aloud while gargling and thereby develops strong resistance against *sore throats* (chapter 1); and the technique of hugging an *asthma* patient from behind, to raise the diaphragm, thereby stopping an asthmatic attack (chapter 9); the easy method of healing the dentist's *skin rash* through the technique of clearing the nerves to his digestive organs (chapter 5); and the simple manner of helping the librarian's distressing *headaches* by showing her how to hold a card in front of her eyes to strengthen peripheral vision (chapter 1).

The wonderfully uncomplicated way to help *appendicitis* by rolling the flesh of the thigh around the thigh-bone (chapter 3); the way to reach the *hard-of-hearing* by removing sludge from the ear ossicles with a simple, self-done technique (chapter 1); the very effective and natural method of helping *spinal disc* problems by tipping back the pelvis and separating the vertebrae to permit the slipped disc to work its way back (chapter 3).

This volume also has many answers that are ridiculously simple, and yet effective and *natural,* to so many other problems that they cannot all be mentioned here. An easy way to clear the sinuses; a simple test for nerve pressures, and a way to correct them; an almost effortless way to ease nervous tension at home; a splendidly effective way to help sexual inadequacy, and on and on. And all of them will be *natural healing answers.* They will accord with the natural needs of the living organism. They will be programs that have been proved useful *in some degree* to all varieties of sick persons, whatever the labels applied to their ailments happened to be.

In short, the purpose of this volume is to show you *how to by-pass the doctor* in many health situations. How to be able to by-pass any kind of doctor safely—that's the aim of this book. How to do things—truly good and helpful things for the human system, without any doctor's help at all.

There is enough in this one book that you are now holding in your hands to enable you to manage almost all but the very gravest illnesses entirely by yourself, and do it exceedingly well. This is a book dedicated to the purpose of teaching you, in simple steps, how to *regain* your health and how to *maintain* your health.

Putting it another way, since nearly everyone nowadays is sick to some extent, this is a book with forty years of experience back of it, to show you how you can personally *un-sick* yourself.

Gall bladders, heart strains, crystals in the kidneys, breathing difficulties, fatigue, rheumatic syndromes, nervous tension, hernias, chronic diarrhea—whatever you have, or in whatever part of the body you happen to have it—somewhere in this volume, there is some good, straight help for you. Why can we be so sure? Because of the way we planned this book to be of the most specific help to you.

The "architecture" of this volume is to start at the head and give readers the answers to problems that affect them in that area: the cranium and scalp and hair; the eyes, the ears, the ailments of the nose, throat, sinuses, mouth, drooping lips, sagging skin of the neck, and so forth. From there, we proceed all the way down the body.

What is your personal health need? During my 40 years of practice, seeing many thousands of people, I have quite probably dealt with your kind of problem many times. And now, through the *Missing Health Link* method, with which you can help yourself and by-pass the doctors, you are ready to begin the program of rejuvenating yourself with a miracle body tune-up. Just look up the answers in this book that apply to you.

THE POWER THAT CREATED YOU
CAN ALSO HEAL YOU

Perhaps it should be mentioned that aside from owning this book there is no further expense or cost. I am not going to rush you out to buy things. No drugs, no costly apparatus. The power to cure you is in the body itself. That power which *created you* can also *heal you.* It's in the nervous system. The nervous system directs the healing, the repair of damaged cells, the functions of all of your body.

It is by way of your body's *nerve pathways* that all your ailing parts are directed in the healing processes and receive the energy for such healing activities. *The Missing Link* takes this into account and makes it work for you (which most healing methods do not). Living the way we do—against gravity in our perpendicular position, straining and heaving and twisting and falling and getting jolted and jarred—no one can help acquiring at some times in his life *cut-off problems* somewhere, on some *nerve lines,* in which case, the organs served by those lines are deprived of healing power and get sick.

When any nerve is blocked or pinched off in some way, (and in our lives it happens in many ways), the healing and functional power cannot get through to the organ which it serves. That is elemental. All doctors of all branches of the healing arts agree with this, for it accords exactly with basic sciences. But not all doctors pay attention to this or are even trained to do anything about it. *The Missing Health Link* enables you, a lay person, to free almost all such occluded or irritated nerve pathways by yourself. This permits heretofore blocked nerve lines again to transmit the healing life force and the proper functional power to the sick organs without interference.

You can see immediately that this is necessary to health, really vital, and should be attended to in all illnesses. But the real discovery is that this, by itself—great and needful though it is—is not quite sufficient.

THE NEGATIVE INFLUENCE OF
GRAVITY ON OUR HEALTH

Another factor is an essential part of *The Missing Health Link.* Because we all live against gravity we all pay a daily toll for doing so.

Thus, in addition to our simple home program of unblocking all pinched nerve pathways, to allow the healing power to get through to our sick organs, we must do something to counteract the daily down-pull of gravity strains on our organs, (fallen stomach, drooping eyelids, sagging colon, prolapsed uterus, varicose veins, fallen arches, weak diaphragm, and so forth). In developing *The Missing Link* I took this into account also and evolved an easy little program that you can follow at home every day.

Please note this—it is of utmost importance. Unless we have a program for doing something about this, with a proper way to *counteract the gravity strains on our organs,* it is in my considered judgment impossible to get wholly well and stay well.

MY SIMPLE THREE-STEP
PROGRAM FOR YOUR HEALTH

Surely there have been enough health systems, methods, therapies. But still you ail and complain. The other methods have just not had *The Missing Health Link;* what they missed was the development of a simple three-pronged program that any sensible person could follow at home. Why *three*-pronged? Because it is not enough merely to balance your body chemistry. With the thousands of very best drugs listed in the United States Pharmacopeia and the National Formulary, if they were enough everybody would be well by now. (As one very wise philosophical researcher once asked: If drugs cure, why does anyone die except of old age?) Changing and improving your blood chemistry is important, but it is only a single step. To change one's body chemistry, the profession of natural hygiene has the world's best and simplest method, as we will explain in the various chapters of this book.

Step No. 2 is still missing. Along with detoxifying your bloodstream in the easy way here set forth, one must know how to get rid of accumulated nerve pressures which prevent the free transmission of healing and functional power to ailing organs—while the organs thus deprived remain sick until they are again served their needed quota of nerve impulses. The way to do this, by yourself, has been developed in my *Missing Link* program. It's so very easy to do, and you can do it at home.

Now there is still No. 3, the step that every method of healing known to me has been lacking. Reverse the gravitational down-pressure on our every organ and vessel and tissue cell. And we have developed a way *this can be done* perfectly in a few minutes of daily attention to our *Missing Link* health program.

I do not wish to labor this point. But it must be obvious to you that with all our fine hospitals and doctors and research centers, *something must have been missing* or you would have been helped. The entire demonstrable truth is that never before has anyone discovered and evolved *The Method*—The Missing Link method of employing the body's own *Miracles for Tuning Up the Sick* and rejuvenating their health. There must always be a first time. The world existed for many years before there was a first time to discover that the earth was round, despite such brainy men as Plato and especially Aristotle. Now there is a truly first time for managing health problems *completely* and properly. Until now the *Link* to tuning up the body and rejuvenating its health has been *Missing.*

HOW TO MAKE THE MOST OF YOUR BODY'S NATURAL HEALING POWERS

What is presented here has already been carefully researched and used on hundreds of cases. *What others have done in reaching better health, you can do* (unless your ailment is irreversible). Our young people, who are intelligently concerned with adverse ecological conditions, are here given a program whereby they can survive despite a polluted atmosphere. Our older people will find in this volume a treasure-house of aids for their geriatric, or just "plain old age," ailments. Case histories described in this book are true. Only the names of persons have been changed to protect the persons' identities.

After 40 years of researching The Missing Link method presented here, and developing and *testing* the link that's been missing in other known doctoring systems, I urge this book upon you, all of you everywhere who are ill, or too stout or too lean, or lost and frightened and exhausted, in order to *pinpoint your* ailment and show you *what to do and how to do it.*

I believe that we have here the long-hoped-for way to health. The very best way whereby those who are *sick of being sick* may tune up and rejuvenate. Rejuvenate *yourself!*—by physiologically directing the use of your own healing power! Use the body's *natural* resident healing power—a power that repairs damaged cells anywhere in the body *if* reachable through clear nerve pathways, and here you are shown how.

Happy rejuvenation to you! As you regain your health and maintain it by means of this book, write me your comments if you wish.

Marsh Morrison, D.C., Ph. C., F.I.C.C.

ACKNOWLEDGEMENTS

I acknowledge deep gratitude to the following persons whose guidance and encouragement, more than that of any others, helped bring this book to birth in its present form:

STANLEY RAPP, former president of Healing Arts Skills, Inc., and original editor of "The Marsh Morrison International Reports," who showed me how to reduce complex subject material to such non-technical writing that even the least-schooled lay person could understand and benefit from it.

HANA HELLER MORRISON, who lovingly but relentlessly did the detective work in ferreting out of the manuscript all solecisms and typographical errors, insisting all the while that "the purchaser of this book must receive at least as much benefit from consulting it as he would receive from a few private consultations in office practice."

Contents

**Doctor Morrison's
Miracle Body Tune-Up
for Rejuvenated Health**

CHAPTER ONE

How to Tune Up and Rejuvenate the Organs of the Head and Neck

Special Note to the Reader:

The specific aids for *specific conditions* in this chapter are best supplemented with the general programs in this book for improving your *general health.* To tune up the body and rejuvenate your health, the best plan offered is *The Missing Health Link* program which shows you how to:

A — Improve the *mechanics* of your body by ridding yourself of nerve pressures and postural distortions . . . .

B — Improve the *chemistry* of your body by easy, sure detoxifying and blood-purifying steps . . . .

C — Compensate for the daily down-strain on your organs by means of proper counter-gravitational drills.

The valuable self-help measures in this chapter will always work better if you couple them with upgrading the general health by means of *The Missing Health Link* program. This is summarized for you in chapter 12 under the *Glossary.*

It's a curious thing. After seeing thousands of patients for forty years, the wonder to me is not that people die. The wonder is that they keep on living with so much the matter with them. From head to toe, everything can get out of order in the body, and often does.

So here at this book's outset, I'm going to start at the top and go down, pinpointing the ailments that can beset you and *showing you what you can do about them.*

If we're going to start at the top, let's make it the very top—the head and scalp. There, some people have alopecia, or loss of hair. If that's your trouble, you will find in the following pages some specific things to do that may help you greatly.

Then there are ear conditions known as tinnitus, and loss of hearing. And eye problems called astigmatism, myopia, and other visual defects. For all these, you will find in this chapter self-help programs of the greatest possible benefit. Still going downward, I'll give you very helpful measures for nasal obstruction and sinus congestions; also for mouth corners that droop or wrinkle; exactly what to do for a tendency toward sore throats, and how to help sagging skin of the neck area. So—let us begin.

THE HEAD AND SCALP

It's remarkable how one remembers the unusual cases of a busy practice, especially those with a lot of human interest. Whenever I hear that women are the vain sex, I remember the strange Mr. John Lucas. He was a popular bandleader who came within an inch of a head-on collision with a truck one night, or in the wee hours of the morning, while returning from an engagement with his orchestra. This frightened him so that rivulets of perspiration poured out of him. In the morning he awoke to find tufts of hair in his bed. They had fallen out during the night. *He had alopecia.*

Well, this handsome man looked a mess and spent the next few years hunting a cure for his baldness and his spotty, weird appearance. His money dwindled and he had to mortgage his home. So-called experts in European capitals couldn't do a thing. The poor man became a recluse. He never allowed himself to be seen with head uncovered, always wearing a cap down to his ears. I was writing a newspaper health column at the time and Mr. Lucas read something I'd written about the galea of the scalp. He came in to see me, cap down to the ears in the waiting room.

I explained to him about the galea, a membrane under the hair which often thickens in adult life, especially in men. This membrane holds together the muscles of the forehead and those of the back of the head, the occiput. When it gets thick, the blood finds it harder to get through to the hair follicles and supply nourishment for hair growth. The first thing I instructed him to do was try thinning down the membrane, then improve the nerve supply to the head and scalp.

What to Do for Baldness,
Alopecia, Falling Hair

"There's an operation for this, John," I told him, "and its purpose is to scrape down the membrane surgically. It isn't always successful, however, and it's pretty costly." He knew about this from an "expert" in Europe and argued against it."But you can do this very often all by yourself," I explained. "Just hold the flat of your left hand firmly against your forehead. Then sweep your right hand backward over the scalp, trying to stretch it. The contact of the right hand on the scalp is very tight and hard. The backward movements are swift and quite forceful. In this way, anchoring the membrane with the left hand on the forehead, you stretch and thin it out with your right."

I instructed him to do this twenty times, two or three times a day. The enthusiastic Mr. Lucas did it all day long. I'd already explained to him that nobody ever gets bald except right over the place where the galea lies underneath; this membrane does not extend to the temples or back of the head and there's never any hair loss there (barring a rare disease, *alopecia universalis*), but only on top of the head, right over the galea. In addition to this technique for stretching the galea, I instructed him to get into the knee-chest position quite often in order to reverse the gravity flow. Also to do the "primordial walk" for general health improvement. And, for special benefits, the "Head-Lift Drill" to insure better nerve supply to the hair—all of which *Missing Link* procedures are explained in chapters 10, 11 and 12.

Now the curious, human interest side of it. In about four months Mr. Lucas came into the office, full of excitement. "Look, Dr. Morrison!" he fairly shouted. He bent his head and pointed to a thin, fine growth of new hair. This growing process continued apace until he looked like a hippie. When I suggested that he get a haircut, it made him angry.

"How can you be so cruel?" he demanded. "Here it's taken me years to get back my hair and you want it shorn!"

But eventually he did cut it to decent length. Being a showman, however, he had photographers present for the occasion "to preserve it in its purity for posterity." For many years, I owned and treasured a photo he'd given me. It showed *His Hairy Lordship* sitting in a barber chair getting his first haircut in years.

THE EARS

Many people suffer from a loss of hearing. Others have a condition called *tinnitus*. If you do not know what this is, you should be glad. If hissing sounds were always pestering you, or you had a roaring or whistling in the ears, you'd have heard the word tinnitus applied to you. In many years of dealing with this and researching the problem, I have discovered some causes and reasons for this category of ailments.

I clearly recall the elderly man who entered my office at the end of a busy day. He was hard of hearing; and I was already tired from examining and treating many patients. But he cupped his hand to the "good" ear and made me expend lots of energy making him hear me. Suddenly an idea hit me. I'd just examined an emphysema case and was wearing my stethoscope. Impulsively I stuck the ear-pieces of the stethoscope into the patients's ears, then spoke through the sensitive diaphragm of the instrument in quiet, easy tones. His eyes glistened, for he heard every word with no effort at all.

"So this is what you fellers listen to people with!" he chuckled. "Now I've finally got to listen through one too—and just wait till I tell 'em."

(Afterward, in teaching seminars throughout the U.S. and Canada, I taught other chiropractors in my classes to use this technique; and thereafter they saved their strength by talking to hard-of-hearing cases through stethoscopes in the patients' ears rather than their own.)

Hard of Hearing . . .
Roaring and Hissing Ears . . .
Tinnitus

It was important to explain to this elderly patient what probably caused his hearing loss, and what he could about it. First of all, therefore, I told him about the ossicles. These are three little bones behind the eardrum which act like tiny tuning forks. They vibrate and *refine the sounds* that come at us raw through the outer ear. But in our civilized mode of living we customarily consume more mucus-forming foods than the system can handle. For some reason, not clearly understood, the excess mucus has an affinity for lodging in these tiny bones and forming a kind of sludge there. This has the consistency of toothpaste. Naturally, such sludge interferes with the free vibration of the ossicles and the hearing becomes fuzzy instead of clear. The bones that are supposed to refine the sounds are half-glued together by the mucus and cannot do their work. Therefore the fuzzy sounds; or the hissing, whistling or roaring noises as the excess mucus sticks and unsticks the ossicles.

Four Steps to Get Rid of Hearing Problems

There are several really good aids for this condition that can be done at home. Of first importance, the nerve supply to the ears must get there without interference. We turn and twist our necks so much that we suffer "cricks" which are actually nerve-root compressions. They block the free transmission of nerve impulses to various organs—the ears in this case. (If ear "experts" tell you that no pinched nerve in the neck can affect hearing, refer them to the *rami communicantes*.) Thus the Head-Lift Drill which is explained fully in chapters 10, 11 and 12 cannot be overdone. Besides this, for reverse circulatory help, one should lie face down crosswise on a bed with the head hanging loosely downward. This stretches the neck area, decompresses the discs between the vertebrae and often releases important nerve impingements. Tinnitus and hard-of-hearing cases should rest in this position twice a day for 15 minutes at a time. The mere weight of the head alone, as it hangs down in a relaxed way, is often enough to help ear problems.

Besides the Head-Lift Drill, which ear cases ought to do conscientiously every day (1.)—and the neck-stretching relaxing program given in the foregoing paragraph (2.)—there is the important third step of avoiding *mucus-forming foods*. People with hearing problems should be aware of the foods which are known to form mucus. They are: butter, cream (both sweet and sour), all cheese except cottage, meat fats, lard, oils, salt, sugar, and even fat-bearing vegetables such as avocados. Milk is not mucus-forming if skimmed; it's the cream content that does the harm.

Foods Which Form Mucus
and Foods Which Dissolve Mucus

Contrariwise, however, there's the important matter of consuming a plenitude of foods which are known to be *mucus solvents*. They tend to dissolve the resident mucus accumulations in the system.

Mucus solvents are all the citrus fruits and all the berries, plus one or two others. Lemons, grapefruits, limes, oranges, tomatoes, pineapple, strawberries, blueberries and all the other berries.

How to Loosen Ear Sludge by Yourself . . .

To add to the above, I must add a fourth step which is an almost miracle-working technique for you. By means of this, you may loosen the "toothpaste" sludge in the ossicles of the ears. Sit down and grasp your earlobe with thumb and forefinger. Stretch it downward. This down-stretch of the earlobe opens the canal. Now, while holding the lobe down at full stretch, jerk it *outward.* While stretching the earlobe down, you see, you jerk it with a short quick snap *straight out to the side.* It is not a powerful jerk, but a quick one. The earlobe, as it is being pulled down, is jerked outward on the level of the ear.

You may hear a clicking sound as you do this. This occurs as the sludge is freed. At once you will hear better. Also there will be a warmth in the ear area for the next 20 minutes or so because of the new circulation. The buzzing, hissing or roaring noises that were so irritating are now gone or markedly reduced. Do this once a day, not more often. Overdoing this technique may irritate the ear.

THE EYES

Miss Alice Younger was a librarian who used her eyes too much in artificial light. Also, like most of us, all the work with her eyes was done *straight front.* The animal sees in a complete arc. But we human beings stupidly do everything only in front of us. We read what's in front of us. We sew, watch television, typewrite, knit, walk and talk with our eyes fixed frontwards. This pulls the eyeballs "out-of-round" and causes the inflowing rays of light to converge wrongly inside the eyes, and we need glasses to make the rays converge at the right spot.

Alice suffered from distressing headaches and astigmatism. At times, half the head and one eye and half the jaw hurt severely, a real migraine involvement. Her side vision was almost totally lacking, for never in her life had she exercised the muscles of peripheral vision and what are called the muscles of accommodation. I told her what to do—easy things that anyone who reads this can do to improve the eyes mightily. She was intelligent and followed instructions. Not only did her headaches leave, but suddenly she needed new glasses because the old ones didn't seem to work for some reason. The oculist gave her the surprise of her life. "Quite strange," he said to her. "Most people need stronger lenses with passing time. Yours require less diopters of correction. Must be that somehow they got stronger and better all by themselves." This was why her glasses suddenly gave her a fit; they'd become too much for her, for now she required less help.

How to Correct Visual Defects:
Astigmatism . . . Myopia . . . Some Migraine
Headaches Which Are Referable to the Eyes

These were my instructions to Miss Younger:

When riding in a car as a passenger, not as a driver, reach into the glove compartment for a folded map or card and hold it in front of your eyes. This will shut out your central vision. It will force you to see only with your side-vision faculties. You will note the passing trees and poles or houses, seeing them with side vision only as the card or map obstructs the front vision. Soon your eyes will get tired from this unaccustomed use of peripheral muscles. To ease and rest them, close the lids tightly and squeeze them together quite hard. This forces the blood out of the capillaries. Now open them with a fluttering, blinking motion. This permits the capillaries to expand and new fresh blood nutrition rushes in. By thus squeezing and opening with a flutter several times you set up a kind of blood-pumping action in the eye areas and provide blood nutrition.

For the muscles of accommodation, Alice was told to hold a forefinger in front of her face and look at it without staring at it. There are three great faults in human vision: to stare at things; failing to roll the eyes in their sockets; not using our side vision. By holding one finger in front of her and *not staring* at it but kind of etching all of it (fingernail, knuckles, etc.) with the eyes blinking relaxedly, she was learning a valuable lesson. Now, looking but not staring, she was to move the finger out to arm's length and back to the face several times. In and out, in and out. This forced her to accommodate to various distances, exercising the muscles of accommodation.

One more drill for Miss Younger. With eyes closed, she was to imagine a huge clock and stretch her eyeballs in all directions, *rotating the eyes within their own sockets,* and with the added benefit that meanwhile they were *bathed in their own lubricating fluid.* Thus, within closed lids, she stretched the eyes to an imaginary 12 o'clock as far up as possible, then 3 o'clock way out to the right, 6 o'clock far down below her feet, then 9 o'clock far out to the left.

She did this several times, then reversed the circle. The eyes were thus stretched until she was somewhat tired, whereupon, as before, she gave them a complete rest by squeezing the lids tightly and opening them with a flutter.

The "Primordial Walk" and *Head-Lift* Induces Better Nerve Supply to the Eyes

All the foregoing were *specific* aids for the eyes. But experience has taught me that with conditions of the eyes the general health must nearly always be improved also. To achieve this, the young lady was told to do those valuable "Primordial Walk" and Head-Lift and Knee-Chest drills that are given in the *Glossary*, chapter 12. They did much to correct the interfering nerve pressures which had been forcing her eyes to function on deprived nerve-supply rations. The strain of this, I was reasonably convinced, had brought on her severe headaches and migraine syndrome—now happily gone.

THE NOSE

Proper breathing is essential to health because it is *not bread but breath* that is the staff of life. If you are a mouth breather, it may be due to several things: deviated septum, redundant cartilage, adenoids, polypi (growths). No matter what, you know that you have some kind of obstruction that interferes with good easy breathing. Even if you are not a mouth breather, there may be times when you would enjoy having nasal passages through which you can draw your breath more satisfactorily. In these times of poor ecology standards, the pollutants often clog our nostrils and we seek relief.

Self-Help for Nasal Obstructions

It is unbelievable how little research has been done in this area of nasal obstructions. Notwithstanding that many people suffer from them, it was only recently that a Soviet scientist concluded 30 years of investigation of the subject. Now at last we can offer a way to help clear the nasal passages of obstructions.

There are three tiny muscles affecting the nose that we almost never use. Not being exercised, they are weak. But if we learn how to exercise them a bit they will respond and get strong. When they are strong, it was discovered, they can dilate the nostrils and widen the breathing passages and give us relief.

In the doctoring business it seems that the smaller the bodily organ or part, the longer its name. That tiny little nothing of a muscle, for example, that dilates the nostril is called *levator labii superioris alaeque nasi.* Ridiculous, isn't it? Maybe it's purposely done to enable us doctors to charge big fees for our alleged knowledge.

What you do to strengthen the three very weak little muscles is as follows. Lie flat on your back and *think* of widening the wings of the nose. It's as much a mental exercise as a physical one. Concentrate on making the nostrils wider. Hold your thumb and forefinger lightly on each side of the nose and feel them dilate. With concentration you gain control again, says the scientists who discovered it, and he's right. After a while, you can just make your nostrils dilate at will. The tiny muscle is strong again, as any muscle gets strong when it is exercised.

That takes care of the first of the three muscles involved. Now, in similar fashion, *concentrate* on raising the tip of the nose. *Lift the tip* toward your forehead. This takes concentration also, but it is easier than the first. Now think of lowering the tip of the nose toward your chin. *Pull that tip down.* You'll find it easy to do after a few tries.

Upon retiring, do each of these muscle workouts 20 times or so. You'll note with surprise that the nasal obstructions have diminished, for your breathing is much easier. You can do this anytime at all besides at bedtime. With doing, it gets easier each time.

THE SINUSES

On each side of the nose there is a sinus which is called the maxillary sinus, as distinguished from the other sinuses of the body. When the maxillary sinuses (or cavities) get congested with pus, mucus, clotted accumulations of bodily wastes, they cause severe pain. One's equilibrium is offside, the head seems to be splitting, every bone cries with pain.

The Simple Technique for Ridding Yourself of Sinus Pains

Mrs. Archibald Blank, a distinguished lady within the British sense of the word, for she was of noble English extraction, suffered what she called "the tortures of the bloody damned" because of frequent sinus attacks. Her visits to the specialist consisted of his forcing a tube through the bony channel (Antrum of Highmore) and sucking out the collected debris. This of course accumulated again and again, for nothing was done to prevent the further piling up of waste matter, and she suffered her attacks again and again. When she came to me she was desperate. I put her on *The Missing Link* program for improving her general health, as given in this volume, and especially insisted that she abstain from eating mucus-forming foods while consuming a lot of mucus-solvent foods, as given on page 28.

"But meanwhile," she hammered at me. "Please give me something to take *meanwhile* for the attacks—until the other program takes effect."

Temporary relief is usually easy, really. This is what I told the lady to do—and it gave her vast relief every time.

> With the cushiony fronts of your thumbs touch the outer corners of your lips. Slide them upward for about an inch and you'll be under the protruding cheekbones. Push up on those cheekbones. Now, while pushing up, slide inward toward the nose and lift as you slide. Your thumbs under the cheekbone fit as though they were under a shelf. Lifting this shelf you slide in toward the nose. Where the cheekbone and the nose join, that is where you lift extra hard. It may be painful right there. You may hear a little clicking sound as you lift with vigor where the bone joins the nose. Almost at once your sinuses have opened, the sinus headache lessens, your breathing is free.

This valuable home remedy for sinus congestion can be done with fair frequency—say twice a day. Nighttime is a good time. Overdoing this at first may be irritating. This is a *meanwhile* aid, not a cure. It is for relief, when needed. For more solid help the general health must be improved, as set forth in the *Missing Link* programs of this book.

THE THROAT

In some families, every time one gets a cold he also suffers a sore throat that hangs on and on. It appears to be a genetic inheritance. Sometimes it's a family trait to get rheumatic ailments if they get sick at all; for others weak lungs or heart problems "run in the family." If you have a throat weakness, it is now known that there's an unbelievably practical and easy way to help you.

What you must do is simplicity itself. Just gargle and pronounce the vowels *aloud* while you gargle. It does not matter what you gargle with. Plain water is fine. Or use lemon juice with it, or bear oil or goose grease, for that matter, if you want to. But the idea is to pronounce in a loud voice A . . . E . . . I . . . O . . . U. In doing this *while the water is gurgling around in your throat,* you must use the muscles that are weak. By using them you make them strong. With strong throat muscles you have the power and the resistance to ward off sore throats. The really remarkable discovery was this: You just cannot help strengthening the weak throat muscles if you say the vowels while gargling because, just to keep from swallowing the nasty stuff, you must give the muscles a workout.

THE THYROID

Those who have visible goiters are very distressed. They are forever seeking help, and now there is help of a kind to offer. In the first place, of course, the nerve supply to the two lobes and isthmus of the thyroid gland must be free to transmit the required Life Force impulses. Thus the Head-Lift Drill given in chapter 11 is of utmost importance. This applies to exophthalmic or *inward* goiter as well as to the outward kind. The counter-gravitational programs summarized in the Glossary (chapter 12) are also enormously valuable here.

Foods which contain organic iodine are of great value. Fresh pineapple leads here. Also useful are tomatoes, kelp, garlic and barley. Vitamin E enables us to "make do" with less oxygen, for which reason goiter cases need this essence of the wheat germ.

But recently another matter has been discovered. This is that there are foods which might be called "goitrogenic," which means goiter-*inducing*. These are the lentils and legumes. So, along with the positive programs for the thyroid problem case that we mention here (daily Head-Lift Drill, counter-gravitational programs such as knee-chest position, "primordial walk," etc.), it might be well to forego the consumption of such nitrogenous foods as beans and peas.

CHAPTER TWO

How to Rejuvenate Yourself Quickly with "Missing Health Link" Techniques

Borrowing a phrase from the foot specialists, when your arms (like your feet) hurt, you hurt all over. Also, when you have emphysema, hardly a moment is worth living. Fighting for every breath is no fun; but a way to achieve greater breathing capacity can be a joy forever. And when the heart is poor you live with constant apprehension. When will my last moment be, that is the ever-recurring question.

Now, however, we have new techniques for all this that tie in with our *Missing Link* researches. In the pages just ahead in this chapter, we have definite, very specific steps by which you can ease and eliminate arm and shoulder pains. And a remarkable way by which you can test yourself for emphysema (do you really have it or was it a mis-diagnosis?), plus an effective plan for building up a stronger breathing apparatus in your body. All this, besides valuable heart-improvement techniques (with even more of this in chapter 4) await you here.

WHAT TO DO FOR ARM AND SHOULDER PAINS

Mrs. George Fabian was a recent widow who suffered from harrowing pains in the arms and shoulders. Her husband had been an eager insurance broker, one of those high achievers who never sold less than a million dollars' worth of policies a year. The widow attributed his unceasing tension to her trouble, claiming it aggravated the pains. Different specialists had named the condition brachial neuritis, frozen shoulder, bursitis. I had long ago discovered the surprising truth that it didn't make much difference as to labels. The treatment for all of them—amazingly!—was very nearly the same, and equally effective.

5 Steps to Getting Rid of Pains in Arms and Shoulders

What I told this elderly lady to do diminished her pains and then eliminated them altogether. The same steps that she was given to follow will probably also eliminate your arm and shoulder pains, barring the rarest exceptions. Here is the program. It is a 5-step, nearly foolproof aid to shoulder and upper-arm neuritis and bursitis.

Step One

First regulate the matter of food intake so as to eliminate irritants that might continually nip and pick on the nerve ends and tissues of the arm and bursae. The patient readily saw the wisdom of this, but expressed surprise that all of this was not told to her before. Her instructions were to eliminate spicy foods of all kinds; eliminate alcohol, carbonated drinks and all ice-cold items. Of great importance was the elimination from the diet of excess proteins. She was told that the body cannot store proteins as it can starches or fats, and the excess not utilized in any day must decompose in the intestines. When she heard that indol, skatol and phenol (carbolic) acids were formed almost exclusively from protein putrefaction in the intestines, she accepted it at once and kept her protein intake down to two ounces a day.

Steps Two through Five were planned to help the arm-and-shoulder area directly. Throughout the years of watching such cases, I've learned that very often the joint (where the arm and collarbone and shoulderblade come together), is jammed together and needs to be un-jammed.

So Step Two is the trick of rolling a heavy Turkish towel into a cylinder shape and wedging it under the armpit. With this rolled towel high under the armpit as a fulcrum, you let the sore arm hang down and with your good arm's hand grasp the hanging arm at the elbow *and pull it inward.* When your arm is pulled in toward the side of your body, the roll under the axilla widens the joint, forcing it apart. This gives immediate, although not lasting, relief. It is a mechanically correct thing to do. The lady said that instead of popping aspirins into her mouth as blithely as though they were gumdrops, she now "spread out" the joint with this towel trick and enjoyed relief at once.

The Third Step was one that required a broomstick or cane. Holding it with your hands about 14 inches apart, you raise it and place it in back of your neck. Because of pain you must sometimes wiggle it into place. But each time you set the stick in back of your neck it comes easier, for the tissues are separated and the nerve pressure is lifted.

Now, for Step 4, you hold the same stick *palms up* and raise it above the head. Holding the stick above your head at arm's length, you do the "hinge" drill. This means that while the arms are straight up, the *forearms* are hinged backward at the elbows. Thus the forearms go back each time while the arms remain straight up. This stretches the bursa in each arm quite effectively.

(Also, Step 4 has a fringe benefit attached to it. It is a direct and forceful exercise for the triceps of the arms, the very place where the "sagging flesh" of middle age occurs in our arms. The saying is, *what we don't use we lose;* but by use through this exercise the flesh firms up. More about this later in its proper place in the book.)

For the Final Step (No. 5) you just try to hang your entire body "dead weight" from loops attached to a chinning bar or tree limb. A bar in the doorway of your bedroom is perfect. Your wrists slide through the loops and you let the body hang. Just hang loosely. At first you will feel the pull in your shoulders. Then in your elbows. Finally, the pull is felt in the intervertebral discs of your spine (about which we have more to say later), and you are getting enormous benefits out of this for your general health as well as the shoulder area.

As always, this matter of your general health ought to be considered if you are to get permanent pain-free years for the rest of your life. I profoundly hope you do the Head-Lift drill and all the other contra-gravitational drills every day at least to some extent—all these to be found in chapter 12.

HOW TO COPE SUCCESSFULLY WITH YOUR EMPHYSEMA

Do you have emphysema—really have it? Or is it merely a glib snap diagnosis that someone made? These things seem to come in vogues, like women's skirts. I remember 50 years ago when everyone—but *everyone*—needed a "T-and-A" (tonsils and adenoids) operation.

Then everyone had to have his appendix out. Later the vogue changed to gall bladder removals, still later hysterectomy operations. Now if it isn't hiatus hernia that you have, any kind of thoracic problem is likely to be labeled emphysema. Better check up, yourself, on this diagnosis. As the saying goes: "Worrying in advance of an event is like paying interest on a note before it falls due."

How to Tell if You Have Emphysema

Light a kitchen match and hold it about three inches from your *open* mouth. Note that "open" is emphasized. Now, without closing your lips to catch a new breath, blow out the light. Blow it out with the resident air, the air that's in you without drawing in new air. If you have enough residual air in the tiny air sacs of your lungs to extinguish the light, then technically it may be said that you do not have emphysema. Could be that the doctor who called it that was just woofing. Or too busy to run it down, he spat out a quick stylish diagnosis. Anyway, don't worry.

What to Do if You Have Emphysema:
3 Steps

But suppose you do have emphysema. You know the kind of coughing you do, the kind that doesn't want to quit. How can you help build up a breathing apparatus that'll be a more effective mechanism? Fortunately, we have researched a most helpful way.

Mr. Patrick Ignatius Joyce had a severe and long-standing case of emphysema. One day, he coughed so uncontrollably hard that his lower dentures came loose and choked him almost to death. If ever anyone needed to build up a better breathing machine, it was Mr. Joyce. I told him to lie flat on his back and lift his legs alternately with knees locked stiff. As he lifted each leg *with vigor,* he was to blow out most *forcefully* all the air that he could. Then he was to let his leg down slowly and inhale slowly. This is almost always the reverse of how a person wants to breathe in and out; the usual inclination is to draw in the breath as the leg goes up, and let it out as the leg goes down. But this is the way that works. It improves the lungs' *remaining* capacity for operation. The air spaces already broken down cannot, I fear, be regenerated.

Mr. P.I. Joyce was a well-disciplined man and observed the instructions completely. When this first step gave him noticeable improvement, he was enthusiastic for the remaining steps. In his inimitable way he said, "I'm rotten-ripe ready for the rest of it, if you please, sir," rubbing his hands with anticipation. So now I told him to count his exhalations so that they took twice as long as his inhalations. "To strengthen the muscles of breathing," I told him, "you have to exhale under control. Take twice as long letting out your breath as drawing it in. While walking, for example. Note how long it takes you to inhale. Say the count is six. In that case count to 12 while exhaling. Toward the end of the count you'll feel the diaphragm and other muscles tightening. You'll be strengthening them." He understood this perfectly and followed the plan with enormous benefits. One day he said he even felt like hiking again, an urge he hadn't had for years.

Diaphragmatic breathing benefits

The last step in his lung-rehabilitation program was the most important in a general way. It improved the health generally.

"Raise your arms," I instructed. "While keeping them aloft, so that the ribs are separated, open your mouth and pant like a dog. Yes, like a dog. With lips open, do some panting. Do this with the mid-section—that's the strong, important diaphragm—moving in and out. Keep on panting like this until you are vaguely tired in only one place. Yes—tired only in the diaphragm. Right where the ribs in front come up to join the breastbone—feel tiredness there. Do this every day, and especially before retiring every night. That'll reoxygenate the entire body. With more oxygen in the system you detoxify better and enjoy improved health."

Most people suffer from a poor oxygenating capacity. They have conditions known as suboxidation ailments. All such ailments get better *to some extent at least* just by doing this *Diaphragmatic Breathing Drill.*

What time of day is best

A word here about when to do this; what time of day is best. The answer to this is so important that we will be repeating it throughout the book. The best time for drills and exercises is at night. Good as it is to be active in the morning on waking, or at other times, the quarter-hour before retiring is best. That's because the benefits that you derive before bedtime are taken with you *during* the hours spent in bed. It's then that the metabolic processes even out, the repair of damaged cells proceeds. Just before retiring, find the freshest area in your house or outside it, and do the Diaphragmatic Breathing Drill.

Another matter that concerns oxygenation. Here, I address nursing mothers who are smokers: also, I address those who love them. If you care at all about giving that nursing infant a fair chance in life, do not smoke during this period. Traces of nicotine have been found in mother's breast milk a mere half hour after smoking a cigarette. No baby should be subjected to imbibing nicotine during its wee formative months, to say the least.

THE HEART: CORONARY OCCLUSIONS
AND TAPPING YOUR LUNG RESERVES

These days there is much talk about jogging and many people follow the advice to jog a good distance each day. I cannot approve of the practice. Most people do themselves harm rather than good by jogging. It may be fine for some who are very well disciplined. *If* you can pace yourself to take plenty of time getting into jogging, and *if* you can take plenty of time getting out of it, then you are safe.

The rule should be to take three times as long working up to jogging, and then three times as long getting back to the normal pace as you spend in jogging itself. One should first walk, then walk rapidly, then very rapidly. After thus working up to it, he may jog. Same way in reverse.

Follow jogging by very rapid walking, less rapid walking, finally normal activity. But the fact to face is this. Most joggers feel so noble after doing their stint of jogging that they sit down to preen themselves. This is too rapid a change, the heart fails to compensate, and a great many joggers suffer collapse. The Diaphragmatic Breathing Drill given above is a better way to tap your lung reserves.

HOW TO HELP EVEN DIFFICULT CASES OF HEART DISEASE

Mr. Whitney Allen Sprague was a man with a serious heart ailment, truly a cardiac cripple. He had been an outstanding athlete in college. Then he entered the family business and planted himself behind a desk. A top executive, using only his head, he had no physical activity at all. His heart which had become compensatorily enlarged during college football and gymnastics, began to adjust to inactivity and sicken with the change. By the time he was 60, Mr. Sprague was an industrialist with pudgy, biscuit-dough flesh, wheezing when he walked and the victim of coronary heart disease.

His wife had received benefits in my office and brought him to me. It was a difficult case to manage. But exactly for this reason, I think it is justified to state here all the steps which were taken in the management of this case. If the reader is a cardiac, he is not as likely to have heart problems as severe as were Mr. Sprague's. Therefore the remedies and programs that almost completely corrected this man's heart disease will in all likelihood help other cardiac cases *faster and better.*

Heart Cases Are Sometimes Psychologically Hard to Handle

Accordingly, here follows in step-by-step sequence the things Mr. Sprague needed to have said to him, and done for him. The reader will easily pick out the many steps that are exactly tailor-made for himself.

"I'm not here because I want to be," Mr. Sprague opened like a small pouting boy. "To reveal my entire mind to you, Dr. Morrison, I have no faith in either you or the kind of treatments you give."

I felt shocked and decided to help this spoiled man most by using the approach he needed.

"Who in blazes asked for your faith?" I half-growled. "This isn't a religion—it's a physical science. All I'd need *if I took you on* would be your faithful attendance to what I order you to do. Time enough for faith when you see some results in your condition."

He seemed a little taken aback. "Well," he hedged, "it's only that Mrs. Sprague here insisted so much. You helped her and she insisted you might help me. Nagging me is what she really did." He smiled faintly. "But I've already seen the very top men in the field everywhere. Shall I tell you what they said?"

"No; that's the last thing I want to hear. If I listened to all that they said and did for you, since they're such very top experts, I'd be inclined to follow their ways. Then I'd do for you what they did. And fail just as they failed."

"I like that," he said begrudgingly. "Makes sense, all right. All right, let's go. I'm yours."

The Monodiet

"Really?" I said it with doubt. To test him I laid out the program that I needed for him *as a starter.* "Three days of monodiets—hardly any food at all," I said warningly. "Only grapefruit for breakfast."

"But I'm a big-breakfast man," he expostulated. "Sets me up for the day that way. The doctors approved . . . "

"Not for cardiacs," I broke in. "Your heart's already over-burdened, digesting big meals takes too much blood-pumping, I want a physiological rest."

I waited for him to absorb what I'd said. He waited also.

"At breakfast, then, only a fruit meal—citrus fruits at first. All the grapefruit you want, or all the oranges, or even fresh tomatoes or fresh pineapple. But only that one kind of food. The best combination is no combination at all."

"And then?" he asked expectantly.

"Then, after a fruit breakfast you get a starch meal for lunch. A small one. Only bananas or only a baked potato. And in the evening, a protein meal of only a couple of ounces of almonds or other nuts, or a bit of cottage cheese. Your coronaries are mushy with a kind of sludge and other cheeses are forbidden. Also, eggs tend to make more of these plaques in the coronaries, so they're out. No items which induce the production of cholesterol, understand. If you have a potato at noon you must add a couple of tablespoonfuls of polyunsaturated corn oil; see that it's *cold pressed,* for heating destroys the value. With the protein you may have a salad of greens. Greens without seasoning. If preferred, put the greens in a blender and whip up a glassful of liquified greens. The greens are neutral and can be had with any meal. That's all you will have for three days. Agreed?"

He nodded.

"Now where are your medicines?" I tested further. "May I see them—all of them—next time you come?" I took courage in both hands and told him the worst. "I will ask to be allowed to flush them all down the toilet."

"But but the blood-thinning ones? The anti-clot medicines. They're vital."

"I'll give you vitamin E. Wheat germ oil. That's nature's own proper anti-coagulant. Drugs are an assault on the body; we'll try to get the system started manufacturing its own needed ingredients for health and self-repair."

How to Build Auxiliary Arteries
to Take the Load Off Occluded Coronaries

It was time for the next step. To get well, he must be shown how to build up some auxiliary arteries to the stricken portions of his heart; and how to reverse the daily toll of gravity on his heart and other organs. *The Missing Link* program in its entirety is what he had to have: to put his body into mechanical adjustment so that pinched nerves to the heart are free to transmit functional power; to purify his bloodstream by means of a detoxifying program and proper food consumption; and to take the strain off his vital organs by means of some simple counter-gravitational drills that his doctors and all other healing arts specialists appeared to have missed completely.

Heart Cases Need *Some* Activity

"I must give you some exercise to do," I said.

"It'll kill me," he replied apprehensively. "My doctors said . . . " He caught himself, and stopped.

"And some necessary *positions* to assume," I continued. "Resting positions, they'll be, but ones that'll favor good solid rest periods for the heart also. You live against gravity. Now we will reverse that and compensate for the gravitational down-pull on your organs."

He appeared more amenable to reason. I asked him to get down on the floor on his hands and knees. He looked silly doing it, but he did it.

"You know what a sway-back is," I said. "Women complain of it all the time when their lower back curves inward. Now while resting comfortably on your hands and knees, consciously *sway* your lower back. Make it as concave as you can. Think of a horse with a deep, sagging backbone—a hollow-backed, built-in saddle." He did this and seemed to enjoy it. "Now then, I want you to reverse this and *arch* your back. Hump it upward as far as you can. The idea is to have your spinal column go down and up, sway and arch, sway and arch—sway *down* as far as possible, then arch *up* as far as possible."

The industrialist did as he was told. "Say, I enjoy this," he said. "I don't have to wheeze as much; I'm breathing easier." It was, of course, true. In that position, the diaphragm fell more nearly into its correct functional position and breathing was less labored.

Now I told him to lie on his back and raise his legs. "Kick your feet," I instructed. "Think of riding a bicycle with the pedals aloft."

He did it gingerly at first, then somewhat faster. I explained that he had to do this very easy exercise, which did not strain the heart because he was resting on his back and the position was properly counter-gravitational. The purpose was to increase the pulse beat somewhat. Only a little at first. Then, as he felt more like it, he would naturally *want* to do more. He would kick his feet more rapidly; later he'd voluntarily ask for more strenuous movements of his body.

How to Know What "Moderate" Means

"Now listen well," I instructed. "Moderate and regular exercise must be done by all people and especially by cardiac people. The word "regular" we can understand—it means just about the same time every day. But what is meant by 'moderate'? How much is moderate? The answer is this in cardiac cases. When your exercise brings your pulse up from an average 70 per minute to about 110-120 per minute, and *keeps it there for 3 minutes,* your system begins to build auxiliary vessels to the heart. New little arteries start to sprout. They feed blood into the stricken portions of the heart that are not receiving their blood quota because their own regular arteries—the coronaries—are occluded."

I asked the gentleman what exercise he preferred. Ruefully he smiled and said "None." He'd been out of touch with exercise for years; now he was afraid of any of it.

"Very well," I said. "Choose whatever form of movements you can tolerate best. If you prefer swimming, or walking rapidly, or whatever. Lying on your back and kicking your feet in bicycle-riding fashion is acceptable, provided you do it fast enough to increase your pulse rate. The only exercises I would prohibit are the one-sided ones like golf, bowling, even swimming with a side stroke. I insist on movements that require the development of both sides of the body, bilateral exercises rather than unilateral ones. The one-sided activities sometimes induce spinal curvatures or scolioses and create nerve pressures."

After watching him accomplish the Sway-Arch movements and the Bicycle-Aloft exercise, which Mr. Sprague relished greatly to his own surprise, I taught his wife to do the Head-Lift Drill to him, for he was yet too weak to do it for himself.

"A most important vagus nerve to the heart comes down through the neck," I explained. "These daily Head-Lift Drills tend to lift the pressure off all nerves in the neck, thus allowing full Life Force to get through to the organs supplied by such nerves." I paused, wondering how to say the next thing. "Do not permit a neurologist and/or a cardiologist to smile and tell you condescendingly that no nerve pressure in the neck can affect the vagus that supplies the heart. If you must, tell him back condescendingly to trace back all the neurological hookups of *ramus communicans.* We have helped too many cardiacs with this program to allow anyone with mere theory to deter us. After all, they haven't helped you, have they?"

What Sprague Accomplished

Thus far our patient had taken several important steps in the get-well program. Most importantly, they included the *Missing Links* never employed in his case before. The Head-Lift Drill was to free his heart-nerves of pressure. The Sway-Arch movements were to adjust his lower backbone and correct interfering pressures on nerves *directly* leading to his heart from the area of the nape of his back or a bit lower down. The Bicycle-Aloft exercise was a first attempt to increase his pulse-rate and build in new, auxiliary arteries to the damaged portions of his heart. The monodiet and physiological rest were to start detoxifying and purifying his bloodstream, which made heart action easier and the repair of heart damages more nearly possible. Now he needed only a bit of knowledge about reversing the gravitational pull on his viscera, and our patient would be off and away to good health.

I explained that he must rest often during the day in the Knee-Chest position, which reverses the gravitational down-pull and compensates in part for the toll which living against gravity exacts from us. Later, while in the Knee-Chest position, I advised the use of rectal dilatation. This merely consisted of inserting a rectal piece (a vaginal douche piece is very good), and keeping it in the rectum for about 15 minutes. This dilates the anal sphincters and contacts a sympathetic nerve ganglion which can affect most desirably those *organs which are not under control of the will,* the heart included. All one needs to know is to lubricate the rectal piece well with wheat germ oil or K-Y jelly or even Vaseline Petroleum Jelly. Just insert it and leave it there; it cannot go anywhere and get lost in the body.

One Great Way to Oxygenate the Body and Help the Heart

The matter of Diaphragmatic Breathing was now in order. This is one thing the cardiac patient must absolutely do every day without fail. It is meant to strengthen the diaphragm and thereby bring more oxygen to the entire body. I instructed the patient merely to raise his arms, not too high but just enough to separate the rib cage, and breathe with his mid-section. It is panting more than breathing, in a way. The mouth is open, the lips apart, and you pant much as a dog does. The only part of you that moves is the diaphragm; you can see its movements just below the breastbone. This is the strongest muscle in the male body. (The female has one muscle that is even stronger, the uterus.) But in most people, especially cardiacs, this once-powerful muscle has become weak from dis-use.

This was the one thing I found it hardest to get Mr. Sprague to do. Although he had been an outstanding athlete, long years of soft living had made him constitutionally lazy, so to speak. Unlike the

Sway-Arch drill on hands and knees, which he enjoyed because it made his breathing easier at once, holding his hands aloft and panting like a dog was too strenuous, he said. I knew it was untrue; he was just spoiled lazy.

"Look," I finally said to him. "I want to succeed on your case—I don't want to fail. Don't you dare make me fail by not following what I advise you to do. Do we remain on this doctor-patient relationship? Or do we part company and you find yourself somebody who'll let *you* manage the case?"

He knew I meant it, and gave in. And he really listened well, with all the great absorbent intelligence that he had, to the explanation I gave him.

Learning From the Baby How to Breathe

"Observe the baby in its crib," I said to him. "The baby's little tummy goes in and out as it breathes. That's the diaphragm working with each respiration. But when that baby is strong enough to pick himself up and *fight gravity in the upright position,* he forgets to breathe with the diaphragm. His breathing is done with only the upper lobes of his lungs, with the apex of each lung—an apical breather. All the reserve store of valuable residual air in his lower lungs goes unused. Only when a man is a long distance runner and keeps on racing until he reaches his 'second wind,' only then, does he tap his lung reserves and use this residual air. Then he can keep on and on, for the reserve store of air is very great. By doing this Diaphragmatic Breathing drill, which I consider one of the most valuable of all my researches, you will tap your lung reserves and help the heart by releasing more oxygen to the body."

He readily understood that his diaphragm was semi-paralyzed from non-use. He also understood that every muscle in the body strengthens with exercise, and *what you don't use you lose.* Thus, he began raising his arms aloft and panting every available free moment he had. He had known that singers are among the few who are trained to use the diaphragm; that's why their tones are powerful and they can hold a note a long time. I told him about my own lecturing experience. In teaching neurological techniques to my classes of drugless doctors, I spoke for four hours at a stretch, with only a ten-minute recess each hour. This needed the use of the diaphragm. "Note this," I said to him. "If I speak from the throat"—and I made my voice high—"in 20 minutes I will be very tired and also my voice will have no carrying quality, no strength or resonance. So I sink the voice down to the diaphragm"—and here I lowered my voice, breathing with the diaphragm from the lower lobes of my lungs instead of from the apices—"and I can go on for hours while my throat is actually resting."

The great thing for him was to know that this increased his body's oxygenating capacity, and that oxygen burned up toxins in the system. He had read about the need for detoxifying and desired this very much. "Good breathing means better oxidation of bodily wastes," I made clear to him. "This affects all suboxidation conditions such as asthma, hay fever, bronchial congestion, wheezing such as yours. Most of all, with more oxygen in the body the heart works more easily and repairs faster."

His spine was beginning to hump into the round-shouldered state typical of many cardiac sufferers. When I introduced him to the "Dowager's Hump" drill (covered fully in the next chapter under *How to Upgrade the Health and Vitality of the Spine and Backbone*), he went at it with great vigor. His chest began to open, he achieved more heart room in the thorax and his upper spine visibly straightened and looked younger. "Man!" he said to me one day with youthful enthusiasm, "I'm really and truly going through a miracle tune-up. I really am."

The Great Lessons of Good Health

Most important, he at last understood the *Missing Link* idea. "Why did I ever waste all those big fees and all that valuable time with the great big, supposedly eminent, specialists," he argued with me, "when they never even told me any of this?" He became a bit doctorish himself—almost pontifically so. "If you don't have good nerves that are free to transmit power to the organs, you just can't make it. You cannot operate the motor without juice. Then if you don't clear the body's accumulated toxins out of the system, you're self-poisoned with your own wastes—so you just have to give yourself what you call that *physiological rest* in order to spruce up the plumbing and get food-utilization going. And certainly, even with the body both mechanically and chemically revitalized, if you let gravitational forces pull you down without compensating for this with your counter-gravitational positions and drills, why then you can't make it either. If you're always being pulled *down* by gravity, without compensating remedies, how can anyone make it *up* to good health, huh?"

He was almost ready to graduate. He knew the score. It was made clear to him that he could on no account permit himself to eat any kind of bakery goods. The additives and cholesterol-making factors were too dangerous for him. Fats and all sugars were eliminated from the diet, but he was permitted avocado as an occasional natural vegetable fat. Polyunsaturated oils, *cold pressed,* were approved; the three best were corn oil, soya and safflower. Many that claimed to be polyunsaturated were not, I warned him. Hydrogenated fats like lard were strictly forbidden. To supply the natural anti-clot element he took, along with daily counter-gravitational drills and the rest, about 600 units of vitamin E from natural wheat germ oil.

The man who had originally come to sneer was the same man who remained to cheer. He lost weight, his pudginess and biscuit-dough flesh turned for the most part to a trimmed-down and flat muscular abdomen, and he lost his wheeze entirely as the breathing capacity increased. To the delight of himself and family, he actually began to do morning push-ups. Then he recalled that the best time to exercise was at night (and knew *why* this was so), so he also did push-ups before retiring. From such sick beginnings, this represented a truly fine rejuvenation of health.

When I discharged Mr. Sprague as no longer requiring my professional care, he reminded me of his first visit.

"I didn't have faith in you, remember?" he asked.

"Yes," I nodded. "And I told you this wasn't a religion and I didn't need your faith."

"That's when I got faith," he grinned. "When you tongue-lashed me with unassailable logic and rode herd on my impertinence, then I really developed faith in you."

He grew pensive about something, and this turned to anger.

"I'm mad clean through," he said finally. "After all the money I gave to those top doctor-fellows! Not one ever made me do any of your sensible things that I so much needed. No one even gave such things a thought, not a single thought!"

"They missed these things," I soothed. "That's why it is The Missing Link. Since I've evolved it, almost no cardiac has failed to be helped to some degree."

Then he exploded. "They didn't miss one thing, though," he fired at me. "Whenever I mentioned going to other kinds of doctors because they weren't reaching my problem, they never missed smiling at me patronizingly as though I were an idiot and dismissing all of you with a wave of the hand. Grandly dismissing all but their own kind of doctors as absolute *do-nothings.*"

"Well, now you know better. Each protects his own kind. People are forever down on what they're not *up on.*"

"Actually, it's true," he said with a small grin. "That label they hung on you, doctor *do-nothings*. You don't know anything of what *they* practice at all. All you know is how to cure people."

CHAPTER THREE

How You Can Rejuvenate the Health and Vitality of Your Spine and Backbone

I think all of us will agree that we cannot enjoy life unless we bring health back to the back. This chapter will be devoted specifically to the man and woman who has to stop from time to time and say, "Ouch . . . my aching back!"

If you read *and heed* what's here—well, chances are that you will hereafter count back troubles as the least of your worries. We know that the nervous system is the Master System of the entire body. All the other systems are subordinate to it. That is to say, the digestive system, genito-urinary system, circulatory and respiratory and all other systems take their orders and derive their power from the nervous system. And—get this—your spine is the switchboard of the nervous system.

All the messages must go through the spinal cord that's inside the spinal column. If your backbone is out of kilter with a vertebra or two out of normal position, often the nerve lines are blocked and the messages can't get through. In such cases the organs that aren't receiving the messages upon which they depend *get sick because they are deprived of energy and directional signals.* So we've got to show you how to get rid of your lumbago and sciatica, your sacroiliac problems and backaches, your curvatures and swaybacks and the rest. Which is exactly what I will do in the following pages.

A QUICK WAY TO REVITALIZE THE TRUNK

In the previous chapter I set forth the self-help techniques for getting rid of arm and shoulder pains that related to the neck. But sometimes the arm miseries and shoulder discomforts come from below the neck. If they stem from the area of the nape of the neck, or the shoulder blades, here are three simple tests that you can make.

Test for Trouble in Upper Spinal Column

First, can you throw a baseball overhand? Addressing the ladies, can you throw a ball the way a man does—*overhand?* Next, can you reach around your back and touch the vertebrae between your shoulder blades? Finally, place the hand of one arm on the shoulder of the opposite side and raise and lower the elbow of the arm that's crossed over. If one or all of these movements produce discomfort or severe pain, your upper spine may need help—the kind of help we will give you right after this next test.

Test for Trouble in the Spine of the Neck

Now sit in a chair and look straight front. With your trunk still and perfectly quiet, rotate the head as far as you can. The idea is to turn the neck—without jerking the head—as far as it will go with reasonable comfort. In order to know how far you can turn in this test, get a fix on some object behind you out of the corner of your eyes. If someone is helping you or watching you make this test, he, or she, can tell you how far you are able to turn your head. But if you do it all by yourself, fix on an object that is farthest away—so that later you'll be able to tell how much farther you can actually see.

Now the object and point of the test is this. *If* you can see farther in one direction than in the other, there is probably something wrong in the spine of your neck. Put another way, if you can turn your neck farther on one side than the other, one vertebra, or even more than one in the neck, may be out of its correct normal position. If this is the case, do a series of Head-Lift Drills and thus lift the head off the neck. (See chapter 11.) This tends to separate the vertebrae and give them a chance, and room, to get back where they belong. When they are in their proper place they *cannot and do not pinch nerves* and give pain. In that case, you can turn freely in both directions. To prove that the magic Head-Lift Drill gave you immediate improvement, turn your head and get a fix in back of you after doing a few. You will find that you can see quite a lot *beyond* the object you fixed as your farthest point before doing the Head-Lifts. All of which proves the important thing you have done: you have un-blocked nerve pressure areas all by yourself. You have made it possible for the free transmission of nerve impulses to areas that were heretofore deprived of power for functional activities. You have induced a miracle, really the body's miracle, and given yourself a fast tune-up just by this one simple technique.

All right, the test for the upper spinal column and the test for the spine of the neck have shown, let's say, that you have some trouble there. This calls for a self-help technique to help every vertebra in your upper backbone (for often the inability to turn your head equally far is due to trouble below the nape of the neck).

How to Help Get Rid of Round Shoulders, Hump-Back, Curvature

Ninety-five percent of all arm and shoulder troubles will be spotted by you, all by yourself, with the above tests. In addition to the trick of rolling a Turkish towel under your armpit and stretching apart the jammed-together joint at the arm socket, as given in the preceding chapter, here's another technique to make results doubly sure. Many people develop a stooped, forward-hunched position at the nape of the neck. This is variously called round shoulders, spinal slouch, hump-back posture. What it is, let's face it, is a curvature of the spine. It may not be severe or serious, but it is a vertebral curvature—a kyphosis in technical parlance.

Did you ever hear of "dowager's hump"? Well, it's the same thing—what the over-rich, underworked, socialite ladies are supposed to dread so much. But they needn't. If it has not yet gone very far, we have the perfect corrective program for it, one that will at the same time help your arms and shoulder discomforts.

Simply clasp your hands behind your back with the *palms touching.* Now roll your elbows inward. Try to make the points of the elbows touch each other. As you do this, a remarkable thing happens. Every vertebra of the upper spine that had been leaning forward like a Tower of Pisa *straightens up.* Your shoulders square back as you give a nice stretch to the bursa of each arm at the same time. And, as a bonus, your pectoral muscles get a workout which makes for improved breast and chest development. All this happens merely by clasping the hands behind you with palms touching, then vigorously rolling the arms and elbows inward. It works! Do it many times a day, and especially before retiring.

HOW TO HELP A SKINNY FLAT-CHESTED CONDITION

Loretta Kinzer was a very tall and very thin young woman—a "spindly scarecrow" is what she called herself. Never married, but indulged by her well-to-do parents as an only daughter of near-thirty, she'd been everywhere trying to get well and get some flesh on her bones. Some luminaries in the doctoring profession had called her case glandular; others said it was psychosomatic. I didn't agree with either label, for Loretta had, I found, what almost everyone else has to some degree. She suffered from nerve pressures which prevented full utilization of the nutritious foods she ate. She was given wrongly combined and overcooked "diets" that I thought would have made a well person sick. And no doctor told her about overcoming the toll that gravity down-strains took out of her every day.

Loretta was normally intelligent. All it needed was a little explaining and she understood what she had to do. The counter-gravitational drills that the reader will find in chapters 10, 11 and 12 of this volume were a joy to do; they revitalized her and gave her pep for the first time in years. But when I gave her this "Dowager's Hump" thing to do—well, that sent her into high altitude. As she clasped her hands behind her back with both palms touching and rolled her elbows inward, she saw her shoulders come up and square out. She looked in the mirror and saw her upper backbone come out of its stoop and become military straight—"straight as a Georgia pine," she said. And when she saw her chest come out "as a chest should"—that capped everything. Her flat-chested front actually curved.

She began to look like a woman and *feel like one*. She did this drill every day and all day long, it seemed, sometimes until she felt she would fairly drop from weariness. But she flowered out into a lovely young woman and even became an expert diver, with no shame at all about being seen on the high-dive board. It wasn't this drill alone that did it; everything in the program helped make her well. But this, more than any one other item in her program, was the technique for her kyphotic spine—her curvature in the making.

PAIN IN THE MIDDLE PORTION OF YOUR BACKBONE

Now, let's go to another part of your spinal column. What if you have trouble, pain, misery in the middle portion of your backbone; is there a good, workable technique for that? Yes, there most certainly is. Many years ago I researched this self-adjusting technique and have taught it with pride to thousands. It is, in truth, a way by which you can *adjust your own nerve pressures* in most cases. Only in troubles that are very far gone, or already very set in the wrong position, will you need the help of a practitioner. In such cases I advise the services of a properly trained chiropractor *as a starter;* then you can take it from there and help yourself the rest of the way. And it is so very easy to do!

How You Can Adjust Your Own Spine with This Valuable Technique

Whereas the preceding "Dowager's Hump" technique made you tall and straight while releasing pinched nerves and correcting *upper*-spine curvatures, this does a similar thing in the lower spinal column. But does it—and a little more—somewhat differently. The ladies have doubtless taken note that the "Dowager's Hump" drill is a developer of pectoral muscles—better chests and firmer breasts. This technique, which I call the Sway and Arch drill, develops the rib cage and waistline while adjusting the spinal distortions at the same time.

How to Adjust a Swayback Condition

Every woman knows what sway-back is. Every man understands the word also, I think. It means an inward-curve of the small of the back, or the lower portion of the spine. Now I want you to get on your hands and knees. While resting like this on four solid points, *consciously sway your back.* Make it cave in. Make it as hollow as you can, like a horse with a deep built-in saddle in its backbone. Having done this, now *arch your backbone and entire spine upward* with as much vigor as you can. Try to make the middle of the spine go up into a real peak. Now make it go down into a deep sway, and up again into a high arch. Sway and Arch, over and over again. This is incredibly effective.

Some will feel inclined to discount this Sway and Arch technique because it is so simple to do. But it was not simple to discover. I remember the long periods given to researching this area of human need. "How can I get people to adjust themselves?" I kept asking my inner self. I tried several hundred different positions and drills, I suppose. With my knowledge of human structure I knew there had to be a way. When the Sway and Arch technique evolved, it *was* the way. To make use of it is simplicity itself. But finding it was something like Edison's discovery of the incandescent lamp. Making use of what he worked up for us is extraordinarily simple: merely a second to push a button and his efforts are employed to our advantage. But to reach his discovery, Edison had to make several hundred experiments over many researching years.

The Sway and Arch Technique

In this book is the first appearance anywhere in print of my Sway and Arch technique. I must emphasize why it is so very important in your future life, lest you tend to ignore it.

In this position on hands and knees, your backbone is firmly based on four points, two hands and two knees. When you vigorously raise and lower the backbone from this position, you exercise every vertebra between the neck and coccyx (tailbone). Being right now the net result of your lifetime strains and stresses, some vertebrae are likely to be out of position. And you will be exercising them. Especially, you will be exercising the contiguous muscles and ligaments which hold the vertebrae in place.

There are five layers of muscles alone overlapping the spine. More than 120 pairs of intrinsic muscles are attached to the spine, pulling on it. All these muscles get a workout as your spine sways and arches, sways and arches, sways and arches. The attached ligaments also get a workout as you sway and arch, stretching the ligaments and relaxing them in turn. Thus, the malpositioned vertebrae have a chance to work back where they belong. The body tends toward the normal. They will work back into place if possible.

You will be adjusting yourself, and need the professional help of a trained doctor of chiropractic only in unusual cases.

HOW TO HANDLE AND GET RID OF YOUR
OWN LOW-BACK PROBLEMS

From the foregoing you already know some very effective ways to handle neck and upper-back problems, and how to perform your own miracle tune-up for rejuvenated health. But that's for the neck, and the arms and shoulders, and for what is called the in-between spine. What about the lower spine? What about your lumbago and sacroiliac troubles and low backaches? For this most important area of your trunk and spine we do, indeed, have a lot of help for you. *I can, in fact, offer you the best and most amazingly helpful self-applying techniques you ever imagined.*

The Program

First, the pelvis. Those two hip-bones of yours are trouble-makers, did you know it? They're the ones that curve around to form the pelvic bowl. Inside that bowl repose the urinary bladder, and all the genitals of the female, and a lot more. These hip bones are technically named the *innominates*, which means the *no-name* ones. But after years of researching those bones I can give them a name, all right. *The trouble-makers;* that's their rightful name!

The way we all live in an upright state, against gravity, the pelvic bowl loses its correct position and *falls forward.* Those hip bones of yours, meaning the top part where you say you place your hands on your hips, are *more frontward* than they ought to be. Where these hip bones come together in front—at the pubic bone which is just behind the triangle of pubic hair—they're malpositioned backwards. It's as though they've been pushed toward the rear, making the entire pelvic bowl a tipped bowl.

This means that the spine and trunk and all the weight above the pelvis are not resting upon something solid below. Your weight comes down the central trunk and is then supposed to rest on a level cross-beam, the pelvis. This is the platform that holds up everything above it. And if it is tipped forward, then what's upstairs (all the body above) does not rest on any solid platform or support.

**THE SELF-HELP TECHNIQUE
FOR GIVING YOURSELF
A SOLID, HEALTHY BACK**

Our contra-gravity manner of living causes another problem also. The pelvis slips downward in front in most people at some time or another. Every female in the western world who is past the age of adolescence probably has a front-downslipped pelvic problem. This is because she changes from low heels to high, back to low, to high, to low, to high. The high heels tip the pelvis forward and force her to compensate by swaying backward—else she would fall on her face. Then the sandals and flats throw her last joint between the final vertebra and pelvis into quite a different work-load.

This eventually causes the pelvis to slip in front at what is called the tendon of Gracilis. In women of the Orient, this may never happen *if* they wear only flats all their lives. Menfolk, however, also have a front-slipped pelvis 50 percent of the time. If you, Mister Male, have ever jumped off a flight of stoop-steps or high fence and landed flat on your heels, and felt the sharp impact in your lower spine when you landed, then you also have a front-slipped pelvis in all probability.

Now, here is an amazingly effective way to "un-tip" your pelvis. Bring it back into line *right under the spine*, not forward-tipped in front of the body weight. Return it to where it serves as a level platform under the entire body, not a lopsided one.

Valuable Pelvic Back-Tip Drill for All Your Lifetime

Every day of your life, so long as you live against gravity, do this Pelvic Back-Tip drill to keep the pelvis where it belongs—where it supports the spine above. Lie on your back and lift one knee. Lace the fingers of your hands around the knee and press it in toward the shoulder on that side. Do not jerk it, just press it down to the chest and shoulder of that side as far as you can. This works the pelvis *backward* on one side. Now flex the other knee and lift it on top of the chest. With the laced fingers of both hands press (don't jerk) this knee toward the chest and shoulder as far down as you can.

This works the pelvis *backward* on that side. Finally, flex both knees and let them rest in bent position above your chest or abdomen. Placing the cupped fingers of one hand on each kneecap, *spread the knees to the approximate width of the shoulders* and press them both back toward the shoulders as far as possible. This works both sides of the pelvis back where it belongs. It brings the pelvic bowl under the spine, not forward or in front of it.

Repeat this morning and night five times. Most importantly, do it at night just before retiring. The benefits you receive just before bedtime you take with you all night. Doing it five times means the following: pressing back the right knee and then the left knee and then both knees, that's one. Five times is actually five times three moves each. Do this without fail for not only the health of your pelvis and lower back but for the entire organism. By returning your pelvic underpinning to a position where it serves as proper support for your entire spinal column, you energize every vertebra and bring health back to the back (and your whole body as well).

One important note for people with low-back pains. The above is not merely to be done morning and night. During the day, *every time your low back hurts,* get down on a flat surface *somewhere* and do this to stretch back the pelvic structures and give yourself ease—ease being the opposite of dis-ease.

HOW TO KEEP FROM GETTING INTO BACK PROBLEMS
IN THE FUTURE

What is the best thing really to make your back healthfully strong? Many different ways of strengthening the back muscles have been researched and fully tested. The best and most strengthening of all is one that I myself worked out a few years ago. It is simple and easy to do. But if done—honestly done every day—it will make the muscles of the back so strong that nothing short of a head-on collision in a car will ever throw your back out of whack. That or possibly jumping from a three-story window.

Squat Drill

The following little Squat Drill is really a kind of knee-bending thing, but with one great difference. You are not permitted to raise the heels as you squat. You squat as low as you can *on flat feet.* Your feet are not together but about *14 inches apart.* I do not wish to be indelicate, but—forgive me—it's the kind of squat the oldtimers did in the woods when they wanted to have a bowel action.

Now the remainder of this drill is as follows. You rise from the squat with your back as straight as you can. Not with your back leaning forward, for then you would be raising yourself with your thighs and knees—and this is not a leg exercise. It is for the back. As you rise from the squat keep straightening your back. The higher you rise the straighter and farther back your trunk leans.

Note: if you feel that you are going to lose your balance and fall backward, then you're doing this correctly. In such a case, if you feel that you're going to fall backward, the heavy muscles of the back are getting a most wonderful workout.

Warning on Squat Drills

This drill can be overdone. Start with just three squats morning and night, especially at night. To be sure you do not actually lose your balance and fall, do this close to a wall. If you should fall the wall would stop you. I would recommend that every week you increase the squats by one. Do four morning and night next week, then five the following week, and so on. In about six months, when you are up to 20 squats, your back muscles will be so very strong that hardly anything will be able to hurt you.

Something to Remember

As you rise from the squat, keeping the heels flat on the floor, spread your arms for balance and try to make your lower backbone concave, like a sway back. Then you can be sure you are working the right muscles in this drill.

ONE WAY TO HANDLE APPENDICITIS
AT HOME BY YOURSELF

When I was a very young doctor a curious thought struck me. I was attending to an appendicitis case, and happened at the time to be researching the effects of thigh muscles which doctors call adductors and abductors. When I turned the flesh of this patient's thigh outward, the hurting lower right abdomen relaxed and subsided. Whereas the skin had been "tight as a drumhead" over the appendix area (McBurney's point), now it let go. I grasped the thigh again high up, as close to the crotch as I could, and rolled it outward some more. In a little while I could even dig into the erstwhile painful point in the lower right abdomen and elicit hardly any distress. This piqued my curiosity. It resulted in my developing a simple little technique for appendicitis.

A Case History of Chronic Appendicitis

Mr. Dolan was a butcher who for many years had what was diagnosed as a chronic appendicitis. Whenever he ate too much, the pain came to plague him. Always it was at the same spot—the appendix point of the abdomen. Surgery was an off-again, on-again deal with him for years. He was scared stiff of operations.

When he came to the office for another matter in the shoulder blades he offhandedly mentioned his chronic appendicitis, expecting no help there. I taught him how to "abduct" the upper flesh of his right thigh. He found it easy to do and followed instructions.

TECHNIQUE FOR COPING WITH APPENDICITIS

"Here is the thigh abducting technique," I told him. "Just lie on your back with knees drawn up, feet flat on the bed. Then reach down to the right thigh with your right hand and let the fingers of your hand fold over the inner surface of the thigh. Now merely roll the flesh around and up—outward and upward. Let the flesh roll around the thigh bone. It's as though you were turning something on a spit with your open hand. Be light, not forceful. Do this half a dozen times, especially at night."

Mr. Dolan did this faithfully as directed and in a few weeks reported with a grin that "all those tormenting pains have gone bye-bye." It was an easy chore I'd given him. "All I did was lie on my back with the knees up and roll the inside of the right thigh up and out. It was duck soup. I don't think," he said hopefully, "that I'll ever have that surgeon's knife stuck into me now."

I would recommend that everyone with a recurring pain in the lower right quadrant of the belly try this technique. It may not help everyone, but it will help many. I would like you to write me your results, if any; I'd like to keep score.

Note: The foregoing technique often helps a case of sciatica with astounding speed. This happens because the rolling movement on the thigh tends to roll the sciatic nerve into the middle of its notch, away from where the nerve is hurtfully jammed against the bony rim of the sciatic notch. If you have left sciatica, do this with the left thigh. Sciatica itself is covered thoroughly in chapter 8.

WHAT TO DO FOR YOUR SPINAL DISCS

These days many people with back trouble are told they have "a spinal disc." This means that the doctor thinks one or more of the cartilages which separate the vertebrae of your spine are in trouble. It may be a ruptured (herniated) disc. More often it is a slipped or protruding disc, which means that the intervertebral padding of the cartilage has been jarred or worked out of position.

A Simple Diagnosis

I can give you a way I've devised by which you can check up on the doctor, for often the diagnosis is wrong. The doctor may have been too busy to run this trouble down properly, or he may not know enough about spinal structural complications. Anyway, I have seen many cases called "spinal disc syndromes" which were not that at all. So here's what I urge you to do. Go back a page or two to the Squat Drill and try it. If you can squat with the feet 14 inches apart *and not raise your heels*, then it's almost certain you do not have a disc problem. It can be any number of other things, muscular or ligamentous or cartilaginous, but if your disc is not where it belongs you aren't likely to be able to squat *without raising your heels*.

TECHNIQUE FOR SELF-HELPING
YOUR SPINAL DISC PROBLEM

If you do have a genuine disc problem, my advice is: Don't rush into surgery. You will be told that you need a laminectomy or other surgical procedure. Don't hurry into this. The technique that follows may be all that you'll ever need. Lie flat on your back on a hard bed. The bed must be hard enough to act as if it splinted your backbone—gave you the feel of firm, hard pressure (like a splint) behind you. While on your back, raise the knees as in the Pelvic Back-Tip drill a few pages back. It will ease you somewhat just to raise the knees to the chest, if you have a true disc problem. Do first one knee, then the other, and finally both knees pressed (but not jerked) toward the chest and shoulders. This separates every vertebra of the lower spine. Being separated, the slipped disc may be able to work itself back into position. (The body tends toward the normal, remember.)

Various Ways to Help Your Disc Case

But suppose this Pelvic Back-Tip drill only eases but doesn't help. In that case, try phase two of this natural technique. While lying on your back, have someone gently and carefully work a hot water bottle under your lower spine where it hurts so much. Or hot towels, wrung almost dry, do as well. Now, have a pan of cold water handy, water filled with ice cubes for extra cold, and a wash-cloth in it. When the "disc area" has been well heated, withdraw the hot towel or bottle and as quickly as you can apply the cold wash-cloth.

The heat has relaxed the parts. Now, the sudden shock of cold causes the contiguous ligaments and muscles to contract sharply. With a quick contraction, the out-of-place disc is often *pushed* back into place. What's working for you is that the body always tends toward the normal. A splinter in your finger works toward the surface if possible. A cinder is your eye is washed out by your own lacrimal fluid if possible. The disc will slip back into position if possible.

Here is another way—or even an additional way—to help your own disc problem *if* you have it, remembering that many alleged disc things are misdiagnosed. From your position on your back, roll onto your hands and knees in the bed, very gingerly, very carefully and slowly. Once resting on four points, you feel relative ease. Now, again very carefully, do the Sway and Arch drill given earlier in this chapter. You are in position for things to happen when you are thus on your hands and knees.

Sometimes the very first Sway and Arch movement of the lower back is done and there's a click. You hear the disc slip back into place, which may give this clicking sound. If this occurs, remain on your knees but lower the front to the chest and maintain the knee-chest position for a long while. If you have someone at home to help you, here's a booster item of incalculable value. Insert a dilator of some kind into the anal opening while you rest in the knee-chest position. There are Young's Dilators for sale which are very good. If this dilator is unavailable, an ordinary vaginal douche piece is fine. Just lubricate it well with wheat germ oil or white Vaseline Petroleum Jelly or K-Y jelly and insert it for 15 minutes or longer. It has nowhere to go; it cannot get lost anywhere. This procedure contacts an important ganglion of the sympathetic nervous system and induces the best rest of the disc patient's life.

I have witnessed incredible looseness in the way doctors label disc cases. Many patients are told that they have ruptured spinal discs. This is possible, but it seldom happens. The discs slip out of place, yes. But those cartilages between the vertebrae are protected by strong body plates which it would take the force of a collision to break. If broken, it's really a case of herniated disc and it is truly serious. Without the protective plates intact, the inner jelly-like substance can ooze out of the disc and really do harm. In these rare cases, I recommend repair surgery as the only proper solution to the problem; but after surgery I want the patient referred back to me immediately, so I can teach him how to avoid disc problems in future.

ARE YOU LESS TALL THAN YOU WERE YEARS AGO?

How You Can Avoid Getting Shorter
As You Get Older

Most people get shorter as they get older. The cause is in the discs of the spine. Every vertebra of your backbone is protected from rubbing and being irritated by its neighbor by means of an elastic disc which is really a heavy pad of cartilage. Recalling that we humans live against gravity, all the weight of our upper body is constantly weighing down on those discs. Then all the jumping and straining you do pounds down on them further. So they get thinned down with advancing age. But I have a simple way to reverse this disc-compressing tendency. Hang by your hands from a couple of loops. Put up a chinning bar in the doorway and suspend two loops from it—or from a pipe somewhere. Then insert your wrists in the loops and just hang. Hang "dead weight," no straining, no pulling against the loop. Allow the body to sag completely; to hang there like a wrung-out rag doll.

This will de-compress the intervertebral discs better than anything else I know. In fact, it is the only thing that will do it successfully. First, you'll feel the dead-weight hanging pull in your arms, and then in your spinal segments. The vertebrae will tend to separate. When separated, there ensues a widening of the foramen through which the spinal nerves pass out to supply the different organs with Life Force. Thus, what you're doing here is also a kind of self-adjustment for pinched nerves. At the same time, the widened vertebrae also permit more room for the blood vessels to send blood nutrition in and carry waste products away.

Do this often. Do it especially just before retiring, if possible. The value of it will be held by you all night, while your weight is off your feet and the discs are not pounded down counter-gravitationally for the next six or eight hours. This tends to reverse the thinning of the discs and the shortening of your stature. Tell your friends about it. They'll be glad to know.

FOR GOOD HEALTH LEARN HOW TO DO THE "PRIMORDIAL WALK"

As indicated earlier, we live against gravity in an upright position. Our structure shows positively that we were meant to function in a horizontal position. The body works best when it is based on top of a four-point platform—on all fours. But there it is, we will continue living perpendicularly no matter what, for certainly we humans aren't about to start living on all fours. So we must do *something;* something to compensate for the deleterious effects of counter-gravitational living.

That something has been developed and perfected for you. It is *The Primordial Walk.* It is a simple therapy that brings you back to how the body *was,* an activity that for a short time at least enables your organism to operate the way it was constructed to operate. Doing this Primordial Walk for only a few minutes daily is enough. It is enough to give motion and strength to every reachable muscle, tendon, cartilage and tendon of your body. That's quite a lot to have done in just one drill. But it is true.

Get down on all fours and walk around a bit. I said on all *fours*—which means hands and *feet.* People unthinkingly believe that all fours means hands and knees, but it's not true. Unless you are very old or seriously debilitated you can do at least a little primordial walking. The exhilarating effect of this is unbounded, almost. While doing this you are returning to what you were meant to be. A mountain of violations are compensated for in only a few minutes.

Even the aged and run-down can try a little of this "all-fours walk"—primordial because it hearkens back to our beginnings—and gain from it. Quite soon thereafter, even they will feel strengthened by it and wish to do a bit more.

Special Note for All Disc Cases

After you have got rid of your slipped disc torment, you must strengthen the lower spine to avoid a return of your trouble. The Squat Drill a few pages back is the thing to do for the *muscles of the lower back*. This Primordial Walk is the thing to do for an *all-over strengthening* of your bodily structures.

THE NEUTRAL BATH

Now to tell you about the *Neutral Bath* and summarize all these "healthifying" items so that you may have a cohesive pattern to anchor to for new dynamic health. Fill a bathtup with water around 99 degrees Farenheit. If you hang a water thermometer from the sides of your tub, or even an ordinary thermometer, the water magnifies the numbers and you'll see 99 (or even 98) easily.

How to Aid the body
in a Neutral Bath

Your average body temperature is 98.6 degrees. Thus if the water in your tub is around the same—say 98 or 99—you will be taking a *Neutral Bath* when you immerse yourself into it. With the *same temperature outside your body as inside,* a great thing happens. Your body, your framework, all the muscles and tissues that make up the *you* of you, will all let go and relax. Being suspended between equivalent temperatures, inside you and on the outside enveloping you, all that can possibly let go in your body does let go. Everything relaxes that can relax.

To give you something to anchor to, then, let us summarize briefly. First you take a Neutral Bath. If you have to catch a train or plane and have but a few hours of sleep before you, do this for 15 minutes. One quarter-hour in a neutral bath will be the equivalent of several hours' restful sleep because your body lets go so completely when immersed between equivalent temperatures.

Summarizing All the Get-Well Steps
for Your Spine and Back

After the Neutral Bath for fifteen minutes or so, do a few Head-Lift drills. This lifts the head off the neck and tends to separate the vertebrae of the neck, thus adjusting the pinched nerves there that are possible to self-adjust. Following the Head-Lift drills, hang for a little bit in loops strung from a chinning bar, or pipe, or ceiling plank. This separates the intervertebral discs, lifts pressures off nerves. After the Loop-Hang (with body dead weight for best effect), get on your hands and knees (knees this time) and go through that wonderfully great self-adjusting technique we call Sway and Arch.

Remember that all this was done after a neutral bath, with all tissues ideally relaxed from the equivalent temperatures, making best self-adjusting results possible. Now, finally, give yourself a workout with several minutes of the Primordial Walk, and follow it by resting in the Knee-Chest position, which is counter-gravitational. While in the knee-chest rest you may, for huge additional value, insert (or have inserted for you) a well-lubricated rectal dilator and keep it there for 15 minutes.

WHY YOU SHOULD NOT DRIVE WITH YOUR ARM RESTING ON THE WINDOW

One final item. If you have arm pains not traceable to other causes, note how you drive your car. Do you rest your arm almost always on the lower frame of your rolled-down window? Do you drive for long stretches like this?

I have seen professionally traveling salesmen with deeply aggravating arm pains that were caused by nothing more than this. Traveling great distances every day with their arm on the window ledge caused them to curve the upper spine to conform—for the window's bottom level is usually higher than one's shoulder. In time, this caused what we call a scoliosis, and a nerve-pressure at the nape of the neck.

The cure? That was easy. I merely instructed them to drive, even on a hot day when they want the window open, with the *window rolled up* three inches—that's all I did. Having the window three inches above the bottom, they couldn't possibly rest their elbow on the ledge. Nor on the window's top, for that was far too high up for comfort. So I merely got them started by "un-pinching" the existing nerve pressures, gave them counter-gravitational drills like those in this book, and positively forbade them from riding in a car with the left window completely rolled down. In their eyes I was a great doctor. In truth, however, I just wasn't a stupid one.

CHAPTER FOUR

How to Have Rejuvenated Heart Function

We know that heart disease is our nation's No. 1 killer. It's a terrible thing to say. Even more terrible to say is this: the death rate from heart disease is increasing, not decreasing. There is something very wrong here. With all our great laboratories and research centers and modern hospital equipment, why aren't the doctors making headway with heart disease? What are they missing?

In this chapter I have a lot to say about this. Here more than in any other area of human disease there is indeed a *Missing Link.* Things which sick people need in order to get well; things being entirely missed in the usual "doctoring" methods. When the reader has finished reading the pages just ahead, he will know what they are. There will not be any more guesswork! I, for one, am not enthusiastic about heart transplants. Let's rehabilitate the hearts we've got inside our chests *now*—there are ways to do it—and not seek foreign hearts to put inside us! As you will soon see, the body's natural rejection mechanism refuses to accept anyone else's organs anyway; it wants its own.

So if you have a heart problem, or a loved one has cardiac difficulties, read and understand every word that follows. Learn what to do for these ailments yourself. Learn what to avoid doing, too. The valuable self-help items set forth here have been successfully tried and retried. Learning them, you may become an expert in your own right.

WHY YOU MUST AVOID TAKING "SHOTS"

Putting first things first, you must not burden the heart with injections of any kind. After studying several thousand heart cases, I have discovered that all injectibles are an assault on the already weak and overburdened heart.

The body rejects having anything shot into it directly. To be acceptable, what's taken into the body must first be *swallowed.* Then *digested.* Then *liquefied* to an *absorbable* state. By that time it's already in the lower small intestines and your body's natural selectivity is at work. The little blood-sucking vessels there do the selecting job. Note, please. They suck into your bloodstream what the blood needs and wants and can use. What isn't compatible with your individual body chemistry *they reject.* The rejected nutrients pass out of your body as waste by way of the bowels or kidneys. They do *not* enter your bloodstream if they are not naturally consonant with the needs of your body.

Have you understood the above? If you have, you are in possession of an important part of the *Missing Link* in heart cases.

The vogue of giving shots for everything (with great profits to pharmaceutical houses) has gained in favor so much that everyone has been given injections for something at some time. And the busy doctors have entirely *missed* an extremely important physiological factor in their shot-giving enthusiasms. The factor which they've missed for so many years is this: whatever by-passes the human safety-valve known as *natural selectivity* burdens the heart.

Don't By-Pass Natural Selectivity . . .
Your Body's Built-In Safety Valve

Let's spell it out. Your body has an intelligence of its own. Every one of the trillion cells in your body has its own intelligence.That is why the body tends so strongly toward the normal. Give it half a chance and it gets well by itself, doctor or no doctor. Thus, when you eat anything which *may be* good and nutritious for you, it will have to go through several steps of inspection and physiological appraisal. If it happens to be violently poisonous, you'll no sooner swallow it than a reverse persistalsis reflex will set in and you'll run for the bathroom to vomit it up. If it is not so terribly poisonous, it gets swallowed all right; but then it has to pass inspection again after it gets through the valve of the stomach into the intestine, and even if it's just half-way bad for you, the body sets up a diarrhea and it gets pushed out of your system in a hurry. That's *natural selectivity* for you. It's the way in which your system protects itself against the possibility of harmful ingredients getting inside of you.

But what happens if all this wonderful natural selectivity is by-passed by doctors who miss the point and have an injection needle in their eager hands? Whatever they are going to shoot into you may not be exactly what your blood would accept for its own. Since your individual blood chemistry is as peculiarly your own as your fingerprints, the chances of any injected matter being precisely like your own blood-needs and blood-wants are almost nil.

So now you've got the point. If the blood doesn't have any say in selecting, with its own intelligent natural selectivity, what it gets, then it must accept what is injected into it. Good or bad, compatible or not, the blood must make do. In "making do" it throws an enormous burden on the heart. Ergo: heart dysfunctions. More injections, more heart disease. With the rising vogue in shots for everything in the doctor's symptomatology, we have a rising incidence in heart disease.

Now you know. You know what this one researching author-doctor has learned—what he couldn't possibly have learned if he'd been trained to give shots in the modern, conventional, *scientific* way.

HOW JOHN JAY WON OUT WITH HIS VERY BAD HEART

John Jay was a rich and highly placed professional man who had had two massive "coronaries" when I saw him. He was in the audience during a lecture I gave, then came forward and spoke in a low, hardly audible voice. I found him an excitingly intelligent man with brilliant, shining eyes; but like many another brainy man, who was an expert thinker in his own field, he had left to possibly vainglorious and inexpert doctors the thinking that had to do with his own body and health. Thus, he accepted the most "godawful" garbage as good sense, simply because "top doctors" had dispensed it.

THE "GOAT GLAND" MAN

Jay had taken "a youngish damsel to wife" and desired to upgrade his sexual ability. One of his "big top man" doctors had advised that he go to Switzerland and see a world-renowned specialist on "cellular therapy." The idea, he was told, was to have the gonads of a goat injected into him, and then he'd be as "feisty" as a goat in the sex department. (Actually, it's the live testicle substance of a sheep that is used, not a goat at all.) He went to Europe, saw the great specialist, and was a recipient of "cellular" therapy.

It was with pleasure that he told me that the therapy must be highly scientific and extra-wonderful, for even a high churchman had gone and one of our own Presidents also had gone there. He spotted the disapproval in my eyes. "You don't think it's great?" he asked. In reply, I asked him one thing. "How long did the people live after their "shots?" This made him wonder. Then, because he was a clever and outstandingly intelligent man, I let go with both barrels.

"Those are live cells they inject into you, did you know that?" He nodded. "Well, the body rejects any and all live matter from whatever source. When will a bright man like you wake up to a clear physiological truth as patent as that? You see what's happening in heart transplant surgery, don't you? Oh, the whole thing's extraordinarily dramatic, I'll grant you, but it ignores the physiologically evident fact that there's a *rejection mechanism* at work in the body. So anybody's heart but your own gets rejected. Meanwhile, just trying to *force* another person's organ on anyone is an enormous burden on the system and wears it out in a hurry."

He got the point at once. "Do you think that I—my heart—the rejection of those live cells . . . ?"

I saw he couldn't face the thought, couldn't put it into words. So I asked him how long it was after he'd returned from abroad that he had his cardiac upsets. In his case, because he had enjoyed more than ordinary vigor, it took quite a while. He'd gone back for another "booster shot" before the body began to rebel. But that's the way the body operates—wanting it to be otherwise doesn't make it so. We had a very long talk about it. And when we finished this lay person knew some Missing Link factors relating to heart disease that even many of our "top" cardiologists haven't yet researched out.

HOW TO STOP BEING VICTIMIZED BY HEART DISEASE

While attending several thousand cases of heart disease professionally, and observing the astounding rise in coronary occlusion these past 40 years, I've come to some quite definite thoughts about it. Here are some do's and dont's that work, that actually work in reducing the incidence of this dread disease. Let us look at them one by one.

Our cardiologists explain the rise in heart disease by saying that times are tough these days—they're full of tension. *I do not believe a word of it.* Four decades ago it was much tougher for everyone to make a living and the tensions were greater! Now, you can fly and hear soothing radio music and be entertained by television. Then, it was a heart-burdening effort just to get from your house to Aunt Minnie's a hundred miles away. And the work was fierce. There was little to entertain and soothe the nerves and iron out your tensions.

Dr. Paul Dudley White says that when he was graduated from medical college he had never seen a case of coronary occlusion, nor had his colleagues. That was about 60 years ago. Coronary artery disease is not a condition easily missed by a doctor; so it must be concluded that there weren't any cases around. What then happened during the past six decades to make this the country's chief killer?

Dr. Wilfrid Shute, a Canadian cardiologist who has personally attended thousands of heart victims, thinks this is due to taking the wheat germ out of our breadstuffs. Since the *natural anti-clot factor* does in fact reside in the wheat kernel presently extracted by the millers in making white flour, Dr. Shute is right. But he is not right enough. There is something else that is of incalculable importance; something that must be attended to or we cannot reasonably expect any diminution in heart disease.

THE CASE AGAINST "SHOTS"

What that something is that must be attended to is the elimination of shots. All intravenous and intramuscular injections, without exception, are a strain on the organism and a burden on the heart. Please reread how injections by-pass the body's natural selectivity (page 66) and understand this vital point for sure.

In my forty years of serving the sick and observing them with researching eyes, this is an unmistakable theory I've come to. Unfortunately, the theory I've developed about the relationship of the rising incidence of heart disease to the rising vogue of giving shots for everything is not a theory that can be buttoned up by demonstrable fact. But it is one that explains itself physiologically—and scientifically. And in the absence of *any* other sensible, unassailably logical explanation that can be acceptable to the scientifically oriented (and non-brainwashed) person, this one must be given deeply thoughtful consideration.

Let us reword it and make is rememberable. My theory is that heart disease has risen step by step with the rising habit of plunging shots into human beings and by-passing the system's natural selectivity—thus burdening human hearts beyond their capacity to withstand.

The Human Skin Is Not a Pincushion.

Your skin was not made to have foreign matter injected into it.

It is not enough to say that the doctors who inject you with cowpox in order to keep you from developing smallpox are sincere. It is not enough to be sincere; you must also be right. And it is not physiologically right to push *any* disease into the body. The job of doctoring is to take away disease, not put it in. And the theory of giving you a lesser disease (cowpox) in order to keep you from getting the greater disease (smallpox) is still a theory that violates the known physiology of the human bloodstream.

We are not discussing here the toll that human kidneys pay in filtering out the heavy wastes from foreign bodies injected into the bloodstream—nor the rise in renal degenerations possibly attributable to the rising vogue in giving shots. We deal here with the heart and its dysfunctions. And it may be set down that the human heart does not thrive on shots, but suffers from them.

Except for the most extraordinary reasons, it is not good doctoring to give shots. It cannot ever be good doctoring to give a person a disease by way of injections in order to prevent his getting another. It *is* good doctoring to raise one's health to the maximum level where the system naturally resists disease—all disease.

For heart cases, there are many things to do. This matter of giving shots is one ultra-important thing *not* to do.

HOW TO TAKE THE STEPS THAT WORK TO REPAIR A DAMAGED HEART

Now let us look at other heart factors that really work to reduce the incidence of cardiac disease and actually do repair the damaged organ, if it is still reparable.

The Case of Henry Snyder

A case in point is that of Henry Snyder. He owned a service station and could barely trudge along a few steps because of his chest tightness and difficult breathing. He'd already been diagnosed (several ways by different doctors) but I wasn't particularly interested in whether the label was endocarditis, myocarditis, angina pectoris or any other. I *was* interested in knowing that it was his heart. I *was* interested in the nerve supply to that ailing heart; whether the nerves were blocked by interfering pressures or were free to transmit the self-healing Life Force to the organ. And I was profoundly interested in his breathing apparatus—how to improve its capacities and how to oxygenate his whole system better. Everything I was interested in was somehow different from what his "expert top doctors" had concentrated on, so it surprised Mr. Snyder when I outlined a get-well program for him.

Panting with Diaphragm in Upright position

Step One. "Henry, can you raise your arms above your head?" I asked.

"Sure can," he said laconically.

"Now can you separate your lips and breathe in and out kind of vigorously through your open mouth?"

"Easy," he said, doing it at once.

"Now do something else, Henry. Pull in your gut with each breath, and then let it out. I want your midriff to be going in and out as you do this panting style of breathing. It'll be a drill to strengthen your diaphragm and make breathing easier."

He did this and liked it. His breathing improved. That was the first step—getting oxygen into his lungs. It gave him the breath (staff) of life; he was less afraid that every heartbeat would be his last one; he could now detoxify the body.

Panting on Hands and Knees

Step Two. I instructed him to get down on his hands and knees. Resting thus on four points he was back to the "primordial position" and his diaphragm flopped more nearly into its proper place, no longer working against gravity. "Do your panting drill in this position," I advised. It was surprisingly easy to do and he liked it. He turned his head like a contented cocker spaniel and winked at me. "I can do this all day," he said. Exactly this was what I encouraged. "Stay in the horizontal position as long and as often as you can, Henry. You begin to overcome the effects of gravity that way, and everything works better." I told him to hang his head and stretch the long neck muscles, something like the animal does when grazing. This separated the intervertebral discs in his neck, tended to lift pressure off nerves and feed his heart with power-impulses and self-repair energy by way of a direct nerve line to the heart, the pneumogastric.

Sway and Arch

Step Three. There were also nerve pathways to his heart from near the nape of the neck and from between the shoulder blades. So our willing patient was taught to sway his back and then arch it: sway and arch back and forth often and with vigor. He was amazed that he had the energy and breath to do it. Actually, in the four-point position it was easier for him to work his body this way than to be upright, against gravity, and do nothing at all. It was explained that this tended to free his body of nerve pressures in order to allow the self-healing Life Force to flow to his heart and breathing apparatus without interference.

Rest in Knee-Chest Position

When he tired of swaying and arching he was directed to lower to his chest and rest in the knee-chest position for as long as he desired. Thus, in the first three steps, I'd taught him to strengthen his breathing muscles and get energizing oxygen into his body; taught him how to self-treat for pinched nerves which had been preventing the transmission of functional power and repair impulses to his organs; and taught him, in part thus far, how to overcome the toll that living against gravity exacted from him every day. All this was achieved so easily and naturally that I decided to move along.

Riding a Bicycle Upside Down

Step Four. "Do you know how to take your pulse, Henry?" He did, and got an "eighty" rate. That was fast; but considering the extra flab he carried around, it was not unusual. "Now roll over on your back and kick your legs," I counseled. He hadn't done any exercise at all and eyed me disapprovingly. "It's what you need," I said firmly. "On your back now, and ride an upside-down bicycle with a little speed," I urged. This raced his heart *a little*, increasing the pulse a bit. "You are going to do more of this every day and with more speed each time," I told him. "Eventually we'll get your pulse up to about a hundred and ten. Then, if we keep it at that for three minutes, do you know what will happen? New little auxiliary vessels to the heart will start building, and that'll take the load off the coronaries."

How to Help Yourself Even When You Don't Do All the Steps

Step Five. "Like most cardiacs and wheezing breathers, Henry, you're slouching," I pointed out to him. "I'm going to make more room for your heart in that chest of yours with what I call the Dowager's Hump drill." He enjoyed clasping his palms behind his back and rolling the elbows inward, thus raising his chest, strengthening the pectoral muscles and getting every vertebra in his upper spine straightened up. But not everyone is willing to do this vigorous drill. It recalled to mind the over-rich and underworked Quincy McKinnon who just wouldn't do this or anything else I advised—except one thing. He almost devoutly loved doing the Primordial Walk (page 62). For a grown man, he was crazy about walking on all fours, like a child who's wild over a new toy.

"Must be my genetic inheritance," he said joyously, looking up at me from hands and feet—not just hands and knees. "I guess I'm only once or twice removed from my four-legged ancestors."

Ordinarily I'd have made short shrift of this overspoiled man who refused to cooperate with me in anything else I advised him to do. I would never have accepted such a person as a patient, preferring to save my energy and doctoring skills for those who wanted to get well enough to follow my instructions. But members of this stringbean-thin young man's family had been good patients at the office since the stringent depression days. They had supported me in my salad days; now it was up to me to support them. Quincy was the indulged favorite of the family and I'd have alienated many of the clan if I'd refused to help. His suffering from a cardiac problem along with emphysema was really heart-rending.

The Primordial Walk

Step Six. This is the Primordial Walk (see page 62) that our spoiled young man loved doing. It meant walking on all fours for real—not the hands and knees but the hands and *feet*. When I developed and studied this drill, I found that it returned us to our first and elemental and original position as human beings. Thus it somehow put everything in the body back into shape that could still be put back into shape—and, most exciting of all, it appeared to exercise just by itself all the muscles, ligaments, tendons and cartilages of the body. This was what the spoiled Quincy McKinnon truly loved to do on the enormous tree-rich lawns of his country home.

Now here is an explanation which perhaps I ought not give, for some readers might forego all the other steps for regaining their health and do only this one as the young man did. Our tall, very thin and wheezy patient dearly loved prancing around the grasses of his home on hands and feet. In a sense he overdid it. But since he did nothing else by way of exercise, his body (tending toward the normal as is natural for all of us) used this one drill to accomplish miracles.

STRETCH EVERY NECK VERTEBRA TO RELIEVE
NERVE PRESSURES TO THE HEART AND LUNGS

With his head hanging down in the manner of grazing animals, every vertebra of the neck got a stretching, and nerve pressures to the heart and lungs were released when the vertebrae widened. With his upper spine straightened by the back-sweeping shoulders supported by his walking arms, the chest filled out and he gained weight. His muscles and ligaments grew strong. The diaphragm operated from a correct horizontal position and his breathing muscles strengthened remarkably. His thighs and legs (at the calves) filled out. With the heart stronger, the breathing easier and oxygenation better, his appetite became evident for the first time in years and he began to eat well. The Primordial Walk alone made the young man superbly well.

Back now to our service station operator, Henry Snyder. Unlike our exclusive Primordial Walk-only man, this great patient observed all the instructions and did beautifully well. Unlike the other, Henry lost weight and flattened out as he grew strong, his chest discomforts left and he breathed easier. This proved to me that the essential rightness of the *Missing Link* factors in doctoring was such that the same basic get-well rules applied to all still-remediable persons. (The undomesticated animal in its wild habitat is never too fat or too thin. The person who is not yet irreversibly sick can get well without the need of a time-wasting precise diagnosis. His body tends toward the normal and wants to be well. It does not await any doctor's diagnosis —or misdiagnosis—to start its own miracle of rejuvenation when the Missing Link doctoring factors are applied.)

In order that sick people get well *fast*—and without the waste of possibly vital time in hunting down a precise diagnosis—the doctor need only know *where* the trouble is. If the patient points to his heart area, or the liver or neck or back, the doctor of the future who knows the *Missing Link* factors will hunt up the nerve supply to the heart or liver or neck or back. If there are pressures on such nerves (as there are likely to be in our straining and counter-gravity form of living), he will know how to release them. Then the healing power and functional energy will flow to the sick organ without interference. And since the human body tends toward the normal, the ailing part will proceed to get well without a diagnosis—which more often than not is a misdiagnosis, anyway. Then, after the *specific* area has been dealt with, the general *Missing Link* factors are applied in order to upgrade the *general* health, and everything that can be done for a patient will be done.

How the Missing Link Treatment Benefits the Heart

Exactly this was now in order for Henry Snyder. For his specific heart and respiratory ailments he was paying all needful attention and was getting well. Now it required only a few general instructions to improve his all-round health and "catch whatever might not have been caught" in ailments that he hadn't reported, or that he himself wasn't yet aware of, or ailments *in the making* that could be eliminated before they reared their head—which is truly preventive health insurance.

One further word about diagnosis must be said here. Suppose the right area of the body and the exact ailment are not treated, even though the patient points to the heart or liver or whatever. It isn't likely, but let's say it's so. Even then, with all the right *Missing Link* health factors in operation on the body, everything that can still get well will get well. That includes those that have been diagnosed, those misdiagnosed, and those not diagnosed at all.

If you have a rash on your hand it gets well in time, whether a doctor has given it a diagnostic label, or given it a wrong label, or not diagnosed it at all. If the nerve lines are free of interference and you are compensating for gravitational down-pressures on your organs, the natural healing processes work to get you well without waiting for a diagnostic label from the doctor. If you wait while he putters around to get *that,* the sick part may be getting sicker and valuable time may be lost in awaiting a pinpoint diagnosis (often wrong), when the *Missing Link* healing procedures could be working on your body *right now.*

HOW TO APPLY A FEW GENERAL RULES WHICH IMPROVE THE ALL-OVER GENERAL HEALTH

For heart cases the first General Rule was to take a good brand of natural Vitamin E from wheat germ oil, say from 400 to 600 International Units a day. (Within the wheat germ resides the d-alpha tocopherol which acts as nature's own *anti-clot ingredient* and is better than the synthetic anti-coagulant prescribed for heart patients.) This assured the blood's remaining thin and not plugging up the coronaries. It was an easy rule to follow and Mr. Snyder took to it readily. Now we needed to make sure that no further cholesterol-forming foods would be consumed to plug his coronary arteries anew. For this it was necessary also to reduce the man's weight.

Rule Two for Digestive Health

"Henry," I asked, "do you like watermelon?" He nodded, being one who talked but little. "Well, Henry, you can have it for tomorrow's breakfast. Just watermelon."

"I'm used to a lot of breakfast, Doctor," he complained.

"And you can have a lot," I said. "A lot of watermelon. All you want. It'll probably make you urinate a lot too, for it's a great diuretic." His ear was cocked for the rest of the bad news. "And for lunch you can have a ripe banana, or even two. And in the evening take about two ounces of nuts, almonds or cashews, together with as large a salad of green raw vegetables as you can hold—with one tablespoonful of cold-pressed corn oil. That'll be your ticket for a whole week. Nothing else." General Rule the Second was what I had given him. It's the best rule I know to change the blood chemistry, give the digestive organs a little physiological rest, and improve the *general* health, as distinguished from the *specific* ailment we were dealing with.

HOW TO STRENGTHEN THE BREATHING MUSCLES

Meanwhile, our willing and beautifully cooperative patient was doing his daily Primordial Walk which, along with the Panting Diaphragm drill, I consider the best of all health-building drills known to man. But there was yet another thing he had to attend to, for here was a man with breathing difficulties complicating his heart disease.

Rule Three

General Rule the Third, accordingly, was to count his exhalations as he walked, and take twice as long exhaling his breaths as he took inhaling them. It was a game. At first, being weak in this department, he could count only three on inhaling so he took six to exhale. Toward the end of even a mere six-count he could feel his breathing muscles tighten, which was the whole idea. Later he inhaled to the count of ten and controlled the exhalations to a whopping count of twenty. He soon enough learned that letting out the air *under control*—rationing it out—gave him a solid midriff and good lung power.

How to Relax

Also for general health improvement he was taught to take a Neutral Bath, and thus relax his body when overstrained. This consisted merely of immersing himself up to his neck in a bathtub with water at around 99 degrees, much like the body's internal temperature. Thus, with the body suspended between equivalent temperatures, everything that could possibly let go and relax did let go and relax.

Best Way to Strengthen the Lower Back

To strengthen his back and not fall victim to the low back problems of so many people, he was taught to do the Squat Drill, with feet spread 14 inches apart and knee-bending *without lifting his heels.* As he came up from each bend, his back was to straighten, not lean forward, causing him almost to fall backward. This strengthened the muscles of the lower back; its purpose was not to strengthen the knees or thighs. For safety, he was instructed to do the Squat Drill against a wall, or a bit in front of one, so that his fall would be stopped by the wall if he lost his balance.

Knee-Chest Position for Countering Gravity Pull

Without fail he did a little of the Head-Lift each day, and this kept the nerves of his neck free of pressures. Occasionally, while resting in the counter-gravitational Knee-Chest position, he inserted a rectal dilator for the anal sphincters. Since we live against gravity, these sphincters tighten severely, especially in people suffering nervous tension, as though to keep the viscera above from falling out. Dilating the sphincters from time to time is an advisable counter-gravitational *Missing Link* measure; and when done before retiring as Mr. Snyder did, it assures the most restful sleep of one's life.

THE DANGER OF EATING MUCUS-FORMING FOODS

It was essential to stop a habit-pattern that is characteristic of respiratory (and heart) patients: that of overloading on mucus-forming foods. So I said to him sternly, "Henry, you must avoid mucus-forming food." And I laid them out for him. No butter allowed. No sweet cream or sour cream, or preserved cheese of any kind, only cottage cheese occasionally. No meat fats. Never any hamburgers or frankfurters because of the usual 30 percent-or-more fat content. No lard or other hydrogenated fats or oils or greases. No whole milk; it may be used only if the cream content (fat) is removed or skimmed off. Not even peanut oil or olive oil; only corn oil, soya oil and safflower oil permitted *if* cold-pressed, for heat destroys the polyunsaturates' value. And no salt or sugar.

Most of all, regular and moderate exercise is needed to rebuild a weak heart. *Three minutes a day* of a fairly quickened pulse, induced by any two-sided activity you like (never unilateral) is what will do it. Lying on your back and kicking your heels. Bicycle riding. Rowing. Swimming. Walking with vigor, swinging the arms and goose-stepping along with it for chest and arm benefits.

The Programs Which Can Rebuild Your Heart

If you also reoxygenate your body with Diaphragmatic Panting and the Primordial Walk while rebuilding the heart through regular and moderate exercise, the remedial process will work faster and better.

If, in addition, you compensate for living against gravity, and also upgrade your blood chemistry through a physiological fasting rest, followed by a week or two of monodiet, you will make the assurance of health doubly assured. Finally, if by means of the Head-Lift and the Sway and Arch and the Dowager's Hump drills you keep the nerve supply to all your organs free of pressures, then the healing power is sure to get through without interruption. Then, what you have a right to expect *will* happen. The power which created you will also heal you. Barring only long-continued ailments that have become deep-seated and irreversible, the miracle within your body can tune up the system and give you rejuvenated health.

Following the aforementioned program is not solely for rebuilding the heart, nor only for strengthening the breathing capacity and reoxygenating the body, vital as these are. It is a *general* plan also. It is *The Way*—the *best* way—to regain and rejuvenate health on all levels.

CHAPTER FIVE

How to Revitalize Your Digestive System in 20 Days for Rejuvenated Health

This chapter is being written with one purpose in mind—to show you how to improve the performance of your digestive organs. With really good digestion achieved, many other ills and symptoms seem to evaporate away. Today, it is even being discovered that all our skin diseases are at bottom really digestive problems, which will be further explained a few pages later.

If you have had digestive upsets, or serious digestive problems in your life, you have probably reached hopefully for the "remedies" advertised so widely. Heaven knows there have been thousands—all promising help, all eventually failing. Yet you continued reaching for more, because hope beats eternal in the the human breast and the drug industry knows it. Surely at least one of the advertised digestive medicines might have helped, out of so many that you tried. The fact that you didn't get permanent help means there was something missing. That wasn't the route to health. Then what was? Exactly what was the missing link?

That's precisely what we expect to deal with here. So let us get into the meaty middle of your digestive problems, and discuss how to revitalize your digestive system right now.

THE CASE OF THE DENTIST'S DIGESTION

Dr. Harry Kay was a dentist. Like all dentists I have seen professionally, he had a lateral curvature from bending to one side over his patients. Of the 300-odd I must have treated, all had a similar scoliosis, or the beginnings of one, and most of them had digestive problems of one kind or another. Their occupational curvature pinched nerves to the digestive organs and caused this. Sometimes, the nerves being impinged upon by malpositioned vertebrae led to the stomach, the liver, or the pancreas. Harry's problem centered in the stomach.

The saying is that what can't be cured must be endured. This hunched-over, better-than-middle-aged man had accepted his digestive problems as permanent fixtures. His feeling of fullness, his heartburn, the all-day burping and the flatulence were there to stay, he was sure. What brought him to me was a skin ailment.

"I still can't believe I'm here," I recall his telling me that first time. He pointed to his right temple and the silvery-scaled rash that at first looked like psoriasis. "I've been to all the skin specialists I could find, but dermatology hasn't got a thing for me. But a colleague had an itch and rash that he says you, of all people, cleared up for him. So here I am."

"Ain't it a shame," I teased. "Me, of all people!" I examined him and felt sure the digestive and skin ailments were connected. Since he was a dentist, it took some explaining to convince him.

A Simple Test for Nerve Pressures

"Turn your head, without jerking, as far as you can to the right," I said. "Note out of the corner of your eye how far you can see. Now turn as far as you can to the left. You cannot turn equally far in both directions, can you? That's one test. You have some nerve pressures in the neck. Being a dentist, you work with some of the cranial nerves, the facial and trigeminus, and so forth. You know about the pneumogastric. Well, you may not be getting a free flow of digestive power to your digestive organs through that nerve. It may be blocked. This test shows you cannot turn equally far; it reveals one important part of the Missing Link."

When I did a few Head-Lift drills for him (see *Glossary*), he could turn farther and see farther out of the corners of his eyes in each direction. This, all by itself, I explained, released some of the nerve pressures and to some degree stopped interfering with the flow of Life Force to his digestive apparatus.

Dr. Harry was impressed by his instant ability to turn better. I told him that he could do it for himself, and he saw its value at once. Also, he understood what harm nerve pressures could inflict.

"That pneumogastric nerve of yours, for instance," I said. "It feeds functional power and also directional energy, to not only your stomach and liver, but also to your esophagus and pharynx and larynx and heart and lungs."

"What a nerve!" said Dr. Harry. That's all he said. All I was explaining represented a new concept to him and he just wanted to listen.

HOW TO HELP SKIN DISEASES BY IMPROVING YOUR DIGESTIVE POWERS

I placed him on two scales and he weighed more on the left, the side toward which his occupational lateral curvature made him lean. The simple exercise of stretching his short side against a wall every day, trying to reach higher each time, reversed the curvature pull and made sense to him. "Why didn't those other high-and-mighty practitioners advise such a simple and sensible thing as this?" he grumbled. "They charged enough for the nothing they did. All they could do well was knock you 'no-drug' doctors."

The important thing he had to know was that if the digestion was poor the skin sometimes took over in eliminating waste products. It is in fact an eliminative organ; the four ways the body uses to get rid of toxic accumulations are: bowels, kidneys, exhalations *and skin*. If all the digestive organs are up to par they are able to utilize the consumed foods and digest them down fully—to their normal end-products of digestion. But if they cannot digest the consumed foods down all the way, there are undigested accumulations in the system. Then the skin takes over to give a helping hand. The skin is a breathing and sweating organ that controls the thermostat of the body ordinarily, leaving direct elimination to the other three eliminative channels. But when the others can't do it all, it often pitches in to help.

The Skin Is Your Air-Conditioning Unit

"The body has its unique intelligence," I told him. "In our work we counsel that you listen to the wisdom of the body. When undigested wastes accumulate in your system, it's like coal not burning down all the way, but only to clinkers, in a poorly adjusted stove. They have to be cleaned out. Your system just has to clear out the accumulated toxins. Usually, your skin is the wrap-around protective organ that weighs about six pounds and protects everything inside of it. It's in charge of air-conditioning, did you know?

To keep your inside temperature at a certain level, usually 98.6 degrees F., it opens its billion pores and sweats out the excess when it's hot outdoors. It closes the pores so tight that you have goose-flesh when it's cold outdoors. And in a pinch, it even doubles in brass as an extra eliminator when the digestive organs are accumulating clinkers, so to say. That's when you have skin diseases. I have never yet seen a skin ailment in a person with free and uninterrupted nerve supply to all his digestive organs. Clear the nerve pathways. Counteract the force of gravity upon your digestive apparatus. *Improve your digestive powers and you will help your skin ailment."*

Dr. Harry was given a program aimed at his digestive organs. The skin trouble which he came to see me about was ignored. He was told to see to the nerves that fed functional power to his stomach and liver and intestinal tract. He was given counter-gravitational drills to follow. Once explained, they made sense to him and were followed. His wife confided to me that he almost religiously did the Primordial Walk morning and night along the length of their hallway, for I'd told him to do this in the largest room or place in the home. He did the Head-Lift and also the Sway and Arch routines to lift pressures from spinal nerves. And he constructed a chinning bar and had a special pair of soft loops made for his wrists, so he could hang dead weight and allow the spinal discs to de-compress.

WALKING TO "DIGEST" A MEAL

"The doctor has even abandoned his after-dinner strolls," his wife told me. The man had heard or read somewhere that one should take a little walk after a meal "to kind of digest it down." I stopped this nonsense, explaining that the animals naturally and *instinctively* curled up and napped after a meal. This accorded with physiology. The blood is needed in the digestive organs to work on the food after you've eaten; it shouldn't be diverted to the muscles while walking or doing any other physical thing. The professional background of this patient caused him to accept this immediately and he cut his beloved strolls. When he went on a short fast, and then on a week of monodiet living, his digestion came back to, as he said, "the kind of excellence I had when I was a boy with a skin stretched around an appetite." With enthusiasm he pointed to his temple. It was fading away; no silvery scales but only a trace of their having been there. Eventually, even the trace was gone.

THE WAY YOUR ARTHRITIS MAY BE
HOOKED UP WITH YOUR DIGESTION

At about the same time, there came to the office a middle-aged, arthritic lady, Mrs. Lucy Curtis. And in her case, curiously enough, almost the same rules and programs to the letter applied to her arthritis as did to Dr. Harry's skin lesions—they were both digestive problems at bottom.

From the way she moved about, I thought Mrs. Curtis had rheumatoid arthritis but I did not say so. She offered to fill me in on all the doctors she had seen and the various kinds of arthritis it was possible for her to have. It disturbed her a bit, I think, when I said it didn't make much difference to me whether hers was rheumatoid arthritis or atrophic, hypertrophic, osteoarthritis, infectious arthritis or any other kind.

THE ENORMOUS IMPORTANCE OF GETTING OVER-ALL HEALTH

"But surely you treat them all differently," she said accusingly. I shook my head. "In the drug-giving style of doctoring you do, Mrs. Curtis. *If* the doctor can pinpoint the kind of arthritis it is exactly, which is seldom. And *if* he can find an exact drug for it, which is more seldom. And *if* it actually helps the arthritis, which is most seldom of all. But for me, it's enough to know it's in your joints. Then, I want to improve your *over-all health,* and that will include the arthritis also." I took courage in both hands and reminded her of something she'd forgotten. "Why, tell me, didn't all those doctors you have seen, or even one of them, find the exact ailment and the right drug and finally help you, if that method of healing has the answer? Why did you find it necessary to come to me?" It was a cruel barb, but it needed saying because she could then transfer this kind of logical thinking to other sick persons who are lost and frightened and don't know where to turn.

Once her thinking got straight, she was an excellent patient. She had heard that high protein meals were good for one, and this nonsense was abandoned when it was explained how little protein the digestion could actually handle. And that the unused, excess proteins she had been consuming caused indol, skatol and phenol (carbolic) acids in her intestines as the direct result of protein putrefaction. "Oh, that's putrid," she said, horrified; then recognized that her exclamation, "putrid," and putrefaction were the same.

This lady wanted to know most of all what to avoid. Her list was just about the same as that given the dentist for his skin problem. The reason? Both the arthritis and the skin disease stemmed from the body's inability to cook fully (digest) the foods these people consumed. The foods just weren't fully reduced down to their normal end-products. They accumulated in the system. In the dentist's case, the toxic accumulations were thrown onto the skin for elimination. In this arthritic case, the uneliminated waste products were shunted onto the joints—out of the way of active circulations to joint areas where there is hardly any circulation. There they piled up and were labeled arthritis. Really a digestive problem basically.

What to Avoid Eating in Arthritis and Skin Diseases

"You must avoid *overcooking your foods,*" I told her. "Also avoid overeating even what is not overcooked, especially proteins. Foods that are much colder than body temperature, or much hotter, must be erased from your allowable items. The hot drinks or foods irritate and inflame the lining of the esophagus and stomach, and cold foods shock the glands which produce the digestive enzymes, temporarily throwing them out of commission. *Do not drink with your meals.* You need all the digestive fluids your body can manufacture, and drinks only liquefy them; they aren't as potent when thinned down by water or coffee or any fluid. Take your last drink 15 minutes before a meal, and do not take any drinks at all until two hours after a meal. Insofar as you can, avoid the foods that have been processed. If they are nicely packaged or enticingly wrapped, there may be more nutrition in the wrapping than in the 'unfoods' advertised as foods."

The above items to avoid were general rather than specific. For improving her digestive powers *specifically* the foods to avoid are the same for all arthritic conditions and skin ailments. They are:

alcohol	carbonated drinks	saccharin	baked goods
butter	preserved cheeses	hamburgers	frankfurters
lard	flavored yogurt	white sugar	raw eggs
spices	jams and jellies	all meat fats	pickled foods
whole milk	cream, sweet and sour	consommes	sour fruits

In addition to the above, these patients are advised to chew every mouthful down to a liquid state before swallowing. This used to have the word "Fletcherize" attached to it. It meant the extra-fine mastication of each mouthful—no fewer than 30 "chews" before sending it down the gullet. This, it was emphasized, was most especially applicable to starchy foods, because they were started in the digestive process right there in the mouth.

WHY STOMACH SLEEPING IS TO BE AVOIDED

Oddly, both the dentist with his skin ailment and Mrs. Curtis with her arthritis were stomach sleepers. This means that they always rested best (they thought) while sleeping face down, the abdomen in contact with the bed. This had to be stopped and I told them why.

"You just can't sleep on the stomach without having to turn your face far to one side," I explained. "You have to turn just to be able to breathe. And with the head turned like that, every vertebra of the neck is twisted and the nerves coming out between the vertebrae are compressed. With pinched nerves in the neck, remember, it is possible to have any and every disease in the body below, or in the head above."

I knew the dentist was thinking of that pneumogastric nerve that he'd labeled "what a nerve!" and I reminded him of a great fact. "Even though that nerve loops around in the head, Harry, any nerve-root compression in the neck can stop the pneumogastric's functional impulses from getting through to the digestive organs— your stomach and liver—and to the heart and other places. So you must learn to sleep on your right side. Or even on your left side, for the heart isn't that far over to the left to be disturbed. Or sleep on your back if you're not bothered by bad dreams and sexual excitement that way. But definitely not on your stomach."

The Simple Technique of Using a Spool of Thread

He really tried. It kept him awake half the night on his side, disciplining himself to fall asleep that way. But that didn't work either. For no sooner was he asleep than he rolled onto his front. His discouragement was profound. But it needn't have been. I asked him if his wife ever used spools of thread, and if he could bring in an empty used-up spool on his next visit. This he did, and I taped it firmly onto the area of his navel. Thereafter, when he unconsciously rolled over on his stomach, it dug into his middle and woke him up. Within a month, a lifelong habit pattern of stomach sleeping was broken.

I remember how he scratched his head and grew amusedly critical over this. "My neck didn't feel exactly right and I asked the doctors if that had anything to do with sleeping on my stomach," he said.

"Most of them dismissed it out of hand as being even too foolish a thought to occupy my brain. They said the baby sleeps like that, so it must be natural. At that time I hadn't had your explanation that only during the extreme flexibility of infancy is stomach sleeping allowed, and that with later neck-rigidity and limited mobility it is harmful. But you know what? There were a couple of doctors who tried to get me off my stomach."

This interested me enormously. I wanted to know what they did for it.

"Oh, some crazy exercises, and even some medicines," he laughed. "When it didn't work they abandoned the effort and said it wasn't important anyway. 'We're doing everything possible, you know,' they said, 'and nothing seems to reach it.' " Dr. Harry paused, grinning with the recollection. "At that time I'd never considered the unfairness of that statement. Whenever they fail, they tell the patient or his family, 'We're doing everything possible' or 'Everything possible is being done for this case,' when it isn't true at all. If they're not using any other method but their own drug-method, they are certainly not doing *everything* possible. They're doing only what *their* method indicates—not what other methods can do." Dr. Harry's education in the natural way to tune up and rejuvenate health was being completed.

THE 20-DAY PROGRAM FOR DIGESTIVE HEALTH

When you understand that the body manufactures its own drugs or ingredients which it needs for health and self-repair, and that *it always did,* you face the big question of your life. What happened to make the body stop manufacturing all that insulin and adrenalin and the rest? And what can you do to make the body get back to manufacturing what it's supposed to manufacture?

In my own researches which began in the early thirties, the answer to the "what happened?" part of it became luminously clear. Although you were born with the ability to make all the drugs and chemicals your body needed for its various operations, the strain of living against gravity and accumulating nerve pressures which interfered with the transmission of Life Force caused your body to lose its power to manufacture what it needed. The hook-up lines (the nerve pathways) couldn't get through to the manufacturing organs because of pinching blockages on the lines, and so the organs couldn't receive the functional power and directions for their manufacturing duties.

Now to the question: *what can you do about it?* And in answer to that one, my researching years have shown exactly what you must do to make the body get back to manufacturing what it's supposed to manufacture.

COMBINING THE 3-DAY FAST; 7-DAY MONODIET; 3-DAY FAST; 7-DAY RAW FOODS

It takes but 20 days to do this—and it can be achieved. Here is the easy, uncomplicated program.

The first three days are spent in fasting. No food at all, and no water except to quench thirst. And no activities whatever. A complete physiological rest (see *Glossary*). This is followed by a full seven days of the monodiet—only one food at each meal. All you want of that one food. (Some have said that they can still overeat if allowed all they want of one food; they cannot, however, because there is a built-in safety valve here due to disgust with the same single food after one's had his fill of it. It is only when you go into different taste levels that you can overeat. Thus, you can have your fill of macaroni, let's say; but along comes the meat and the new flavors and savors arouse new taste levels. Then you are stuffed to the limit with meat, but you can still be aroused by the taste of ice cream or chocolate pie, etc.) Following the week on the monodiet, another perfect physiological rest by fasting three more days. Finally, a full week of raw foods exclusively: salad greens, whole or blended in a liquefier; solid and satisfying foods such as grapes, avocados, coconuts and bananas; all the fruits and other vegetables you desire, but in the unfired (raw) state. On the theory that man was originally a fruitarian—and only then a vegetarian—and finally, an eater of everything in sight, this plan returns the organism and digestive apparatus to primordial status and enables it to "catch up" with itself.

SUMMARY OF THE 20-DAY PROGRAM

The foregoing plan takes 20 days. During the non-fasting 14 of these 20 days you attend to the other "needfuls." Essentials, really. They are the daily unfailing attention to the activities and drills which un-pinch the nerves to the digestive organs, plus reversing the gravitational strains and stresses on your body. Consult the *Glossary* and do the Head-Lift, the Dowager's Hump, the Sway and Arch, and Diaphragmatic Breathing and Pelvic Back-Tip and the rest. For resting periods the favored position should be the Knee-Chest. For all-round daily workouts it should always be the Primordial Walk. To strengthen the lower back you ought not neglect the Squat Drill. To de-compress the spinal discs *hang from the loops* daily, as explained herein; and from time to time take a Neutral Bath and also 15 minutes of Rectal Dilatation; and on rising in the morning accomplish the transition from the horizontal to vertical by means of the One-Spot Walk (for all of which see the *Glossary*).

Only 20 days. If you are truly in earnest about changing your direction and enjoying health instead of illness, just carve 20 days out of your life and do the above—all the above. You will be grateful you did; for all the tomorrows of your lifetime you'll be glad.

HOW TO PROGRAM YOUR ORDER OF DR. MORRISON'S HEALTH BUILDERS

To borrow a phrase from the great Abraham Maslow ("The Hierarchy of Needs"), and change it a bit, I must answer a question that intelligent patients have often asked since this research came into being. "What is the order of importance to all your *Missing Link* factors?" they want to know. "We are convinced that the various healing arts have had missing elements, or they'd have been able to get ahead instead of behind with major diseases. We are also convinced that you have discovered these vital missing techniques. But, they cannot all be *equally* important. Tell us then, Dr. Morrison, what is the chief *Missing Link* among them, then the next in order of importance, then the *next* next, and so on."

Accordingly, I set forth here what I can best call the *Priority of Needs*. To find the answer in full honesty to this serious query, I asked myself a question—an academic one. "What if you, Marsh Morrison, had time for only one *Missing Link* technique, which would it be?"

The answer was forthcoming at once. Faced with such an unthinkable situation as being able to assure my health through only one activity, I would do the Primordial Walk. I'd do it with energy and frequency. It would exercise everything reachable in me. It would tend also to adjust my spine, lifting pressures off the various nerve pathways—since the body tends toward the normal and awaits only your doing the right thing, giving it half a chance, so to speak.

THE 5-STEP ORDER OF MISSING LINK TUNE-UPS

Some of the other portions of the Missing Link program are almost as important—such as Diaphragmatic Breathing to oxygenate the system—and the Head-Lift to take pressures off vital nerves in the neck—but I'm sure the Primordial Walk would be first choice.

Looking at this another way, assuming that there is a real hierarchy of needs in the quest for health, what are the needs in their order of value? Part of this is academic, anyway, for one can do conscious breathing with the diagram in the Knee-Chest position, thus merging two techniques at the same time. But perhaps it would be most helpful to put the Priority of Needs according to classes rather than techniques. Put that way, they are:

1. *Counter-Gravitational Techniques.* These are the most helpful, and greatest, of all among factors missing in doctoring.

2. *Nerve-Pressure Correction.* Pinched nerves cannot transmit Life Force and functional energy to organs, so correcting nerve pressures should be foremost in doctoring.

3. *Oxygenation Drills.* Strengthening human breathing apparatus is vital to health but has been largely unattended to in most doctoring programs.

4. *Detoxification and Blood Purification.* The easy ways to do this through fasts and monodiets have been missing, but the drugging way, with consequent side-effects, has not.

5. *Nervous Tension.* Great natural techniques to achieve tension releases are available but have been missing in doctoring methods which favor more complex, profitable ways.

CHAPTER SIX

How to Regain the Full Potential of Your Liver, Kidneys, Pancreas, and Gall Bladder for That "Totally Alive" Feeling

More people these days suffer from maladies of the liver and kidneys, and of the gall bladder, than ever before in the history of our nation. Long ago, I discovered what I believe to be the reason for this. Almost everyone in the country consumes far too much of the sugars and starchy foods which overwork the liver to an enormous degree. Almost everyone has at one time or another been "talked into" taking shots, and my researches show a tremendous strain on human kidneys as they filter out the injected protein poisons. And almost everyone eats in such a way as to engorge the gall bladder, congesting the gall bladder duct and thereby blocking the way to "Total Health."

Eating as mentioned above would be enough to cause harm. But when we do this and live against gravity *in addition,* that's an extra jolt to healthful human metabolism. And when we have, besides all this, the accumulation of nerve pressures that everyone gets in our form of living (and which interfere with the transmission of Life Force nerve impulses to the liver, kidneys and gall bladder), then we have ample reason for our day-to-day health problems.

But there is cause for hope. This is because we have not alone found the reasons for our health problems, but the answers to them.

Now we know how to correct most, if not all, liver and kidney and gall bladder ailments. And how to do it *naturally*. Not with expensive doctoring methods (that haven't reached our problems anyway), but with sensible and effective methods, described in this chapter, that you can apply at home.

If you have felt droopy, listless, and lacking the previous vigor you recall you had years ago, then this chapter is for you. If the tubules of your kidneys could stand a thorough cleansing and reinvigorating metabolic lease on life, then here you may learn how to reach your full potential. If you have suffered the profound distress of gall bladder congestion, just ahead of you are pages with advice that may make you feel "totally alive" again!

THE CASE OF THE CHINESE MEDICAL HEART RESEARCHER

Dr. James Lu had come to the United States from Formosa on a heart research grant. I'd met him socially and invited him to visit the office to see what I was doing with cardiac cases. Chain-smoking swiftly as many Orientals do, he told me his special field was investigating new techniques for photographing the insides of the heart.

I noticed that he burped frequently and had a yellowish cast to his eyes. On inquiry, he said he'd gone "completely American" with his love of frankfurters and soda pops, hamburgers and Southern "frieds" and especially beer and pretzels. This caused a great deal of gas formation, enough to give him heart discomfort. When I ventured that his problem might be digestive in origin, he agreed to "have a go at eating only apples for a while—and then only grapes for a while."

James did not like the fasting idea at all; but he'd heard about the pectin in apples and the tartrates in grapes. Rather quickly, the organic pectin in raw apples cleansed him, also giving new strength to the circular intestinal fibers that had gone weak. Meanwhile, his liver rested and, being a self-repairing organ, mended itself all on its own. This surprised the young Chinese, for his medical training taught him to do *something,* and here I was counseling him to "do nothing intelligently."

"I must bring these techniques back with me to Formosa," he said, feeling much improved. There was no more gas and consequently no further gas-pressure transferred against his heart, so the cardiac symptoms subsided. Then he went on grapes for three days and the natural organic sugars so compatibly met his organism's needs that they picked up his energy index at once. He diagnosed himself "entirely cured."

The entire *natural healing approach* was foreign to his medical training and he wanted to absorb all he could about the *Missing Link* factors I had developed. The idea that we all suffered ills because as bipeds we lived against gravity was both fascinating and astounding to him. "It's almost entirely different from what I have been trained to search for in causation of disease," he declared, "but yet it sounds correct." He agreed that right there I might have stumbled onto one major reason "why we do not gain better on heart dysfunctions and mental illness and cancer."

WHY COLD DRINKS HEAT YOU UP

Since our young Chinese friend "dearly loved" his cold beers on our hot days, I mentioned the body's thermogenetic centers to him. "You know," I said, "that anything you consume that's way above the normal human 98.6 degrees temperature must be cooled down to normal body temperature, so your cold beers must be heated up to the rest of the body temperature. Well then, in the process of heating up the beers *all of you* gets heated up in the process!"

We laughed about this. "Charming," he said. "It sounds so very right." The Russians, I pointed out, had caught on to this long ago. On hot days they drink their hot tea, which is so hot the body has to cool it down to normal 98.6—and that cools them down all over.

POTASSIUM-RICH FOODS ARE GOOD FOR PEOPLE . . .
SODIUM-RICH FOODS ARE NOT

He reminded me that when I'd suggested apples for his digestive ills he respected me immediately because of what he'd learned in his own heart research. "Sodium-rich items, like *salt,* are bad for the heart." Foods rich in potassium, they were discovering, were good for the heart. Since fruits were richest of all in this mineral, eating apples for his digestion, which I said might be the cause of his heart problem, appealed to him. Then, when he recognized the value and aptness of the pectin factor in the apples, he knew, he said, that "you non-medical doctors must have much indeed that we medical people do not possess."

He mentioned a case that needed the gall bladder removed by surgery, and I asked how he knew absolutely that surgery was needed. He had never thought to question it. The surgeon had said it was necessary, wasn't that enough? "No," I said. "My years in this profession have taught me to question everything. We have ways to avoid surgery in most cases of common bile duct obstruction and congestion. To ask a surgeon whether you need surgery is like asking a car salesman whether you need a car—or asking insurance people whether or not you ought to buy insurance."

HOW TO AVOID GALL BLADDER SURGERY

An excellent way to clear the bile duct of its clogging debris has been found to be very simple. Just cook up a mess of beet leaves. No one knows why this works. It cannot be explained why there's an affinity between plain boiled beet leaves, not the stems or the beet itself, and the piled-up rubbish in the duct which conveys bile from the gall bladder to the upper intestines.

It's an empirical method, a very simple aid. There's nothing wrong with empirical self-proved methods so long as what you use cannot harm you in any way, and beet leaves certainly can't. So that's one way to help the congested common bile duct naturally: *eating a large portion of plain, boiled, unseasoned beet leaves, and nothing else that day,* customarily does the vital clean-up job for you.

Another way is to immerse oneself in a bathtub of quite hot water, as hot as can be borne. Heat dilates, opens up the body's passages. Many times this also dilates the gall bile duct sufficiently to let the congested matter in the duct work itself through and out into the duodenum section of the intestine.

Along with this, of course, the nerve pressures must be corrected, and in gall bladder ailments there always are nerve impingements to be attended to. By following the techniques in this book's *Glossary* you will have all the aids you usually need.

HOW YOU CAN EASILY CLEAN OUT YOUR KIDNEYS AND BLADDER

Of all the disagreeable and hurtful medical techniques, the urologist's cystoscopic examination ranks way up on top. But there are effective *natural* ways to houseclean your kidneys and urinary bladder. Those who have taken sulfa drugs have run the risk of having harmful crystals accumulate in the kidneys. Those who must rise at night, or urinate often during the day because of body acid concentrates or other irritants, can use a good diuretic that leaves no toxic side-effect problems. Following are my recommendations for home remedies.

Watermelon and Pears

For the bladder, watermelon is the best diuretic (kidneys and bladder flusher) that I've ever used. But if eaten in large gobs it won't do the work. It should be cut into little cubes, say an inch in size, and one of these watermelon cubes should be popped into the mouth at spaced intervals all day long. One cube every 3 to 5 minutes would be about right.

In this way the bladder gets "geared" to the drip-drip, drop-by-drop descent of the watermelon fluid and reacts to it. You will find yourself urinating more than you ever did in your life before. Do not eat or drink anything else that day. If watermelon is out of season, pears may do almost as well. I've found Bartlett pears best. These are also cubed or sliced into small portions and consumed every 3 to 5 minutes all day long.

Raw Beet Juice: How to Drink It

For the kidneys themselves, quite another technique has been found extraordinarily effective. I refer to *raw beet juice,* not beet leaves this time. The beet itself is placed in a juicer raw, and its juice drunk in small spoonfuls throughout the day. Here, curiously, the empirical remedy was discovered because it was observed that over-eager food faddists who guzzled raw beet juice by the tumbler-ful made themselves deathly ill.

Beet juice, when researched, was found to be potent stuff. The body won't take much of it at a time. But when spooned to a person every few minutes all through the day, it helped greatly. No sickness followed. The urine turned red, as did the stools. At times even kidney gravel and sulfa-formed crystals went cascading out over the renal threshhold and were heard hitting the porcelain bowl as they left the body!

How to Drink Beet Juice for Best Results

Ration yourself to 8 ounces of the raw beet juice for the entire day. Nothing else eaten or drunk that day. The hundreds of tiny kidney tubes get the cleansing of their lives. While taking a spoonful of the juice every few minutes, consult the *Glossary* and give yourself additional help by compensating for counter-gravitational living, by correcting nerve pressures, by oxygenating your body anew, and by rest. *Note that these techniques are not cures.* They give relief, they cleanse the congested areas, they start you toward rejuvenated health. But there is no magic. *No single button can be pushed to make you well.* Health is the result of a program, not any single drug or even any single technique I've developed. The special techniques will help you gain health, but *to maintain health* please follow the entire program.

THE UNTOLD STORY OF "SHOTS"
(THE INJECTIONS "THEY" WANT YOU TO TAKE)

Our young medical heart researcher was entranced with most of the foregoing, but could not quite go along with the idea that there was no magic in drugs. Especially shots. Surely shots were not harmful to human welfare. "Look at what they've done to clean up disease," he insisted.

At this time another chiropractor brought a grave cardiac case to me for consultation. It was an interesting history because what had happened to the "cardiac cripple" was what could have happened to any of us. He'd merely ridden a long way on a bus and fallen asleep with his neck in an awkward position. On waking he could hardly turn his neck, and for a year there was "a smallish pain there," as he put it. When heart symptoms developed and he mentioned the neck incident, no cardiologist connected the neck symptoms with the heart problem.

Then the patient, Mr. Gratz, a skillful cabinet maker who'd enjoyed exceptional health before falling asleep on that bus, planned a trip abroad and took the required "shots." This triggered the heart attacks. He barely escaped alive out of his coronary occlusions.

HOW NECK PAINS CAN BE CONNECTED
WITH HEART TROUBLE

Both Dr. Ben——, the referring chiropractor, and my Chinese friend were present but I directed my remarks to the medical man. "Number one in this case," I said to him," is this neck trouble. Not one of your people who specialized in hearts took notice of the nerve pressure in this man's neck that prevented the flow of Life Force to his heart. You must see how vital this is, or all our study of the nervous system is a farce. And number two is the body's own *natural selectivity* that outlaws shots which further burden the heart. Yet shots are given by cardiologists as blithely as they hand out aspirins.

"I say that the nerve pressure right here, in this neck, weakened his heart—and it could have been corrected so easily by the right doctor who knew how. And I say further that the shots themselves nearly killed him when his heart was already weak from inadequate nerve supply."

"But injections can also do very much good," Dr. Lu said. "See how smallpox is nearly wiped out and how polio is presently diminished."

"Yes, and look at the increase in heart disease," Dr. Ben broke in. "And in renal degenerations as the result of having to filter the poisonous mess out of the body."

The patient was of course an interested listener. Now he said his say in the soft, measured tones of the cardiac sufferer.

"I was lucky, actually. My sister's husband was given a shot and died right there in the bed." His lips trembled a little with the fury of recall. "They told me not to go near any chiropractor because their adjustments would kill me. I never heard of anyone dying right there from an adjustment the way my brother-in-law did. But I've since heard about a lot of men dying from shots. So how can they make such unprofessional accusations?"

"Yes," Dr. Ben charged in. "And we chiropractors never yet made a dope fiend out of anyone!"

YOUR BODY'S PROTECTIVE SAFETY VALVE: NATURAL SELECTIVITY

Being a cardiologist himself, and a researcher in the field of the heart, Dr. Lu's eyes opened wide when I presented my theory connecting the increased vogue in giving shots for various maladies with the increased incidence of heart disease. "Do you have a better theory?" I asked. "Sixty years ago there were no coronary occlusions at all. In those six decades, the pharmaceutical firms have talked the doctors into giving shots for everything in the symptomatology. They even put out a booklet once that they mailed to the drug-prescribing profession. The booklet's title was: *How to Build a Lucrative Practice on the Needle.* It set forth the ease with which money could be earned, using injections as the way to earn it. If you had a roomful of patients in the waiting room, and also desired to run off to that bridge game or wrestling match, your nurse could "clear out those 20 waiting patients" by giving them each a shot of B-12, the booklet set forth temptingly. All your fees would be coming in, and the profit would be enormous. (The vials at one time were 20¢ each in dozen lots and the fee for injecting them into human skins was around $7.50.)

"The smallpox vaccine shoots cowpox, which is a disease of the calf, into the bloodstream. How dare professional doctors of any kind give you *any* disease, even on the promise of protecting you (hopefully) from a greater one!" I waited for this to get deep into our friend's consciousness, then went on. "But everywhere in the world where there is good plumbing, good sanitary engineering, good flush toilets to carry off human waste products, there is no more smallpox—shots or no shots. And wherever there is a breakdown in sanitary facilities, smallpox breaks out again regardless of how many shots were given. This happened in the Philippines when it was under American rule and the population received smallpox shots every six months under Army edict. But when good plumbing conditions failed in Rizal, smallpox raged so terribly that the population of Rizal Filipinos suffered the highest smallpox death rate known to man—and all of them were previously injected and re-injected with smallpox vaccine many times. The only ones who escaped the epidemic, it seemed, were those natives who'd been afraid of getting their skin 'pincushioned by the Army' and had run off to hide in the woods when the vaccinator hove in sight. Is it any wonder that now, Dr. Lu, our own government agencies have finally got the idea and no longer require smallpox shots either to go abroad or come back home?"

WHAT POLIO INJECTIONS CONTAIN

Our conversation brought out the salient points that people ought to know for their protection—and that the Chinese ought to take back to his people. First was the point that the body must select *naturally* what it needs, and wants, and can use. This it does by way of the mouth: digesting and absorbing what it can use, and rejecting by way of the eliminative channels what it does not need and cannot use. Every person's blood chemistry is as individual as his fingerprints. It is virtually impossible for any injectible to be exactly like one's own blood chemistry. Therefore, whatever by-passes the organism's natural selectivity by being shot directly into the skin, must be unlike the body's own chemistry to some extent and must be a burden on the heart and kidneys.

"The shots for polio," I offered, "might all by themselves have triggered incalculable heart maladies, considering what goes into them. First the poisoned blood of Rhesus monkeys—who wants that in his bloodstream? Then this sick blood mixed with more than 60 chemicals, and all of it treated with formaldehyde, which is embalming fluid. Can you tell us *physiologically* how this can do anything other than break down human hearts? That polio injection is so strong to take that it can swap symptoms. It can divert what might have been polio to something else. Anything else. You cannot prove that it doesn't. I can prove that heart diseases have risen, and I think it does. No wonder they themselves don't consider it perfect— else why seek an oral shot like the Sabin vaccine?"

WHAT YOU OUGHT TO KNOW ABOUT HEART TRANSPLANTS

Dr. Ben brought up the matter of acupuncture, and Dr. Lu agreed that it ought to be discussed by us. I agreed also—for later. Since Lu was a heart man, first we ought to take our blinders off and have a clearsighted look at transplant heart surgery. Right off, I said that in view of all the known physiological facts and truths—and cutting out all the heroics and dramatics—transplanting the heart was a chimera and a delusion. Well! That started the ball rolling. If looks could kill! The greatest thing in Dr. Lu's field of cardiology, and I waved it aside as though it were nothing. How could I!

"If doctors in all schools of healing took hold of the *Missing Link*, people would be mending the hearts they've got, and not be looking to transplant the hearts of others into their chests." Both Dr. Lu and Dr. Ben considered that carefully. "Just looking at the nerve supply to the heart, which we'll do directly," I added, "and just a silly little simple thing like the Dowager's Hump to make more chest room for a slouching heart patient with insufficient working space—that alone would save more hearts than all your drugs which assault more than they aid. And easy daily compensations for the burden on the heart due to living, and pumping, against gravity. Little compensations like the Knee-Chest position and the Head-Hang over one's bed—and then the vital Primordial Walk. And just doing the extraordinarily easy but very effective Diaphragmatic Breathing to bring life-giving oxygen to the heart. And purifying the heart's blood supply through a bit of fasting, and sensible dieting, and extra-sensible physiological rest that brings the self-healing heart back to its rejuvenated potential—that's how to save the heart you've got!"

WHY THE HUMAN BODY REJECTS OUTSIDE ORGANS

Calling the business of heart surgery a chimera and delusion sounded unforgivable. I had to validate myself professionally.

"The body is known to reject all living cells and organs and matter put into it. Sometimes a kidney transplant will take. But that's because there are two of them, and the other can take over the burden of the work. Even then the natural *rejection mechanism* goes to work and the job doesn't 'take' for long. Corneal transplants can be relatively successful because they are but small parts of the organism and all the rest of the system can work to make this transplant stick—besides which the eyes are very vascular and all the inflowing blood nutrition can help. But when there's only one, as is true with the heart—it's a delusion to expect more than temporary heroics. And dramatics. And kudos for the fancy surgeons.

"That power which created you, that's also the power that can heal you! It lacks only the employment of what's been missing until now. *The Missing Link.* The body tends strongly toward the normal. It *wants* to be well. It heals *itself.* There's life and self-repair power left in your body even when far gone with disease. Just reverse the gravitational down-pull on your organs. Clean up your health-delivering bloodstream. Release from the nerve pathways the interfering pressures which all of us collect in our straining workaday lives. Put the body into mechanical *ease.* That's the opposite of *dis*-ease.

"There is more life in even a dead human being than there is in a living one-cell organism. So I say to sick people, after many years of treating them and observing miracle rejuvenations in otherwise irremediable cases, I say to them, DON'T DESPAIR! Remember that the same power that made you can heal you if it can reach the sick parts. And here we show you how."

HOW TO LIFT OFF NERVE PRESSURES BY YOURSELF

Now I suggested that we look at the nerve supply to the heart and other organs. Our Chinese researcher readily agreed. When I asked, "How can anyone expect Mr. Gratz's heart, for instance, to be normal when the functional nerve impulses can't get through to the heart because of pinched nerves?" he seemed a bit bewildered. He was taught to diagnose the heart condition exactly—if possible. His research was to try and photograph the heart from the inside. "Then what?" I asked. "Suppose you know down to a hairline what's the exact pathology in Mr. Gratz's heart, tell me precisely what you'll do to help him." It would be difficult, he agreed. It would be a matter, then, of finding an exact drug to help the man.

But were there any such exact drugs? And even if there were, how could any drug under heaven lift pressures off nerves to the heart? Could a drug straighten out a low shoulder? Can a pill or injection fix a short leg or a high hip or a spinal curvature?

The researcher then asked the leading question. "How many are there in the world," he wanted to know, "who have the skill to correct nerve pressures of the kind you mention?"

"Everyone in the world if necessary," I answered at once. "I can give you such easy-to-do Head-Lift and Dowager's Hump and Sway and Arch drills to do at home that you—yes you, yourself—can get rid of most if not all the nerve pressures from which you suffer this minute."

HOW LAY PEOPLE CAN ADJUST THEIR OWN VERTEBRAE

I began to demonstrate how the Sway and Arch and the Pelvic Back-Tip, just as examples, tended to adjust the vertebrae into proper alignment. Here Dr. Ben fired a query at me.

Was this ethical? Was it quite right to teach lay people how to adjust themselves? Wasn't it tantamount to teaching people how to abandon their chiropractic doctors?

"Never fear," I assured him. "Teaching them how to adjust themselves will also teach them to think of themselves as machines, as mechanical mechanisms who are subject to mechanical mal-adjustments. They'll know that you chiropractic doctors are the experts—the only doctors trained to adjust the body's mechanical ailments—and they will save you for the complicated, important things. To go to you fellows for every little adjustment that they can be taught to do themselves—well, it's like going to a drug-prescribing doctor to get a band-aid."

Our young doctor of chiropractic was hardly convinced. So I reminded him of what happened years ago, when he was yet too young to appraise it. Television came in and everyone could have movies of a sort in his own home. Surely this would close down every movie house in the country. But what it did was help the motion picture business. "Where Macy goes, Gimbel's follows," I said. "And then it's better for all of them. Teach the people how to get well and be well, that's the needful thing. Then they'll hunt you out for what they just can't cope with themselves."

Dr. Ben thought about this. Dr. Lu wanted to believe it.

"Look," I said. "We're three doctors here, and I think we'll agree that if three things in the body work well—the heart, the breathing mechanism, and the digestion—the rest of the body will also usually work pretty well."

HOW TO ATTEND TO YOUR OWN NERVE SUPPLY
FOR DIGESTION, OXYGENATION AND HEART ACTION

They nodded their heads in agreement. Now I demonstrated the technique of Diaphragmatic Breathing and it convinced them beyond doubt that this alone, so very easy to do, would improve the muscles of breathing. On top of that I demonstrated the Sway and Arch, and they could see the movement of the vertebrae through which passed the nerves to the digestive organs. Such movement, they conceded, could very likely adjust back to normal whatever nerve pressures happened to exist. Now I came face to face with something more difficult: our Chinese researcher's heart area and its nerve supply interferences.

"Turn your head as far as you can to left and right, Dr. Lu," I said, "and note how far you can turn—not far enough, huh?" He appeared surprised that he could turn much farther on his right side than his left. "Now do this Head-Lift," and I did it for him (see *Glossary,* chapter 12). His eyes bugged because at once he could turn farther in both directions and could see, scientifically, that a neck area that had been blocked was now free of interference—free to transmit nerve impulses to whatever organs were served by the nerves traversing that presently-free neck area.

"Now James," I said, addressing the Chinese doctor, "there's a lesson for you in this simple technique—and for everyone you care to teach it to. You know that the chief neurological hook-up with the heart is the vagus nerve. You know that the heart needs the impulses from the vagus, and if deprived of those impulses it just cannot be well. Well, here with merely this technique that I have just shown you, and can teach almost anyone to do for himself, I have made possible a free flow of impulses to the heart where a moment ago the flow of these power-impulses was blocked. The moment you could turn the neck farther, that moment the area through which those impulses must flow down to the heart was opened. Every heart patient can be taught to do this. Every heart patient should be."

THREE EASY VITAL STEPS TO HEALTH

I gave them time to let the whole big idea soak in.

"What *is* it that we know right now about helping this heart?" I asked. "We know three things: how to improve the breathing capacity of the body through the Diaphragmatic Breathing drill. That's one thing. We know how to upgrade the digestive capacity of the body through supplying more Life Force to digestive organs by means of the Sway and Arch technique. That's number two. And we know how to lift off the nerve pressures to the heart by means of the Head-Lift. So there are the three vital things on which the body depends: cardiac function, digestion, oxygenation. When heart patients do these things we've just talked about *plus* counter-gravitational drills and blood purifying techniques, why—you've made the assurance of good natural health doubly sure."

HOW TO HANDLE LIVER CONDITIONS,
DIABETES, AND ORDINARY CONSTIPATION

Our friend the Chinese heart researcher asked if he could bring to me a young lady receptionist from his research center, for he wanted us both to discuss her case. She had, he thought, some kind of liver trouble besides the diabetes which had plagued her since her teens. "Let me see how you go at a patient from the very start," he said. This, in his opinion, would enable him to grasp the non-drugging approach to healing sick bodies better than all the theories and discussions he could think of. "We try to diagnose it right away, but you don't. May I see how you do it then?" he asked.

Since there was no question as to Miss Rosemary's diabetes, we spent little time on that beyond some relevant remarks. The eminent Dr. Alexis Carrel wrote that insulin did not cure anything but only supplied hopefully what the body itself was not able to manufacture.

IS IT NECESSARY TO DIAGNOSE?

"We know," I reminded my friend, "that diabetes is more grave in a young person than in an older one. This is because the pancreas was made to last a lifetime manufacturing insulin. If it breaks down late in life, well, there might be some reason for its wearing out. But to quit being able to manufacture insulin early in life, that's serious. So here we need to apply logic and ask ourselves a logical question. What happened, do you suppose, between the day Rosemary had no diabetes and the day she did? Did her pancreas just impulsively, or capriciously, decide to quit making insulin? Or was it more likely that she had a fall, a jarring impact or twist of some kind in her active, upright manner of living, that brought about pressure on nerves leading to that pancreas? The kind of nerve pressure that prevented the flow of Life Force and functional energy to the pancreas. We must investigate the nerve supply to the pancreas first of all, you see."

I traced out the nerves at her spine and found that two vertebrae were in fact out of position, pinching vital nerves. In addition, Rosemary had discoverable nerve pressures on pathways to her liver.

"Now James, tell me if you think we need to diagnose the way you people do?" I asked him, as I was marking out the involved nerves with a skin-marking pencil. "I could begin treating her right now, just knowing it's her pancreas and liver that are in trouble. How much valuable treatment time would I waste if I had to wait for a precise, pinpointed diagnosis?"

This was a difficult area for Dr. Lu. One cannot shake off in a hurry the training of four years. "How many years have you given to memorizing sets of symptoms in order to be able to give them diagnostic labels? All that label-seeking in order to know what drugs to give—when in fact no drugs can cure, but a system of health might." It was important to me to convince him that we do not actually need to diagnose. If the health of our people depended on exact diagnoses, I pointed out, everyone would die in a hurry because so very few—according to recent medical surveys—were exactly correct. "It's almost impossible for any doctor in his rush-rush way to call it right. You almost have to live with a patient around the clock for a few days to be able to diagnose with precision. No doctor has the time for this, and few patients could afford such exclusive service. You know the rule, James. *Treat the patient, not the condition.* To know the patient, you just about have to live with him, don't you?"

Dr. Lu grew pensive. "Even those in our family that we do live with; do we diagnose them correctly every time?" he mused.

I kept hammering at the central thought. "Take this liver problem of Rosemary's. Does it really make any difference whether it is cirrhosis, or a portal circulation involvement, or hepatitis or anything else that specific? Isn't it enough that I know it's the liver I want to treat? Here are the nerves to the organ, and they're blocked by vertebrae that are out of position and pinching them. We know how to un-pinch the nerves. That'll permit the functional power to get through to the liver once more. And if the liver isn't yet irreversible, it'll get well regardless of what we name *or don't name* the condition."

APPLES AND PAPAYA FOR CONSTIPATION

I showed the young lady how to start herself on a get-well program. It included all sides and factors of the *Missing Link*—all the things the other doctors had missed doing or missed teaching her to do. She was shown the wisdom of attending daily to a few counter-gravitational movements which would compensate for the ills of living against gravity. The Head-Lift and Dowager's Hump and Sway and Arch drills taught her how to keep on adjusting her spine after I gave her an initial start in this direction. As is customary in liver problems, she was also constipated and I asked if she knew where to purchase papayas shipped in from Mexico or Hawaii. A raw apple the last thing at night, followed by half a glass of water, supplied a kind of bolus for the circular muscles of the intestines and assured good bowel evacuations in many cases. The papaya, if available, dug into the undigested, accumulated protein wastes and cleared them out of the system, due to the protein digestive enzyme it contained. The re-oxygenating program was outlined for her also by way of Diaphragmatic Breathing and the other drills—all as outlined in the *Glossary* of this book. It but remained to do something about her diabetes.

This was admittedly difficult. A pronounced diabetic problem was always serious in the young. There was, however, one rather faint ray of hope. It has been discovered that on occasion the diabetic is helped by eating only tomatoes for half a day. At least the need for insulin is eliminated in some cases. The plan is to test oneself and go according to the needs. Canned tomatoes seem to work perfectly well in this plan, often even better than fresh tomatoes for a reason not understood. The diabetic eats only the contents of a can of tomatoes until 2 o'clock in the afternoon. Nothing else. The large can contains only two or three very large tomatoes, but these easily constitute a meal. No salt should be taken. Often, merely eating only tomatoes in this way, daily until 2 o'clock, is enough to eliminate the need for insulin. When done together with the programs here given for contra-gravitational drills, and self-adjustment of the pinched nerves, the chance of success is much enhanced.

IS THERE VALUE IN EATING LIVER FOR ANEMIA?

Miss Rosemary, a thin girl with a wan face and flashing, intelligent eyes, made an observation. We had been discussing her case in front of her. In my own open, non-secretive way with patients I feared that I sometimes offended the Chinese medical researcher, for he'd been trained to have professional discussions out of hearing of those involved. The rule always amused me. "When you think, you control your thoughts; when you speak, your thoughts control you." This meant that so long as you didn't give explanations or opinions to patients, if you were wrong at first you could change your mind and the patient would never know you'd been wrong. (When you think [not speak], you control your thoughts. But if you speak out your opinion, then you have to stick to them [your thoughts control you].) As a result of our free and easy discussion of Rosemary's case in front of her, she came to her keen observation.

"Advertising and brainwashing propaganda can do things, can't they?" she said wanly. "I used to think that the drug-prescribing kind of doctoring was the only kind there was. At least the only *scientific* kind worth noticing—to hear them tell it. But now I learn that there are many doctoring professions that use no drugs at all. Right here, I've learned about chiropractors, and homeopaths who are also medical doctors but hate drugs, and naturopaths, and natural hygienists, and naprapaths and hydrotherapists and such. The things you learn . . . the things you hear that you didn't know!"

MORE QUESTIONS ON LIVER DIET

Because of Rosemary's low energy index, Dr. Lu asked if she might not do well getting appropriable iron and good protein from broiled liver. There was a matter worth discussing, for it could be handled well or badly.

We know that the human liver has at all times about one-third of the body's entire blood it it. If our little lady, Rosemary, weighed 100 pounds she would have something close to two quarts of blood in that liver of hers—about one-thirteenth of the body weight. Animals can be assumed to have the same amount of blood in their liver, I think. And since the "life is in the blood," as the Bible reminds us, an anemic person or a person generally low in energy ought to be able to derive much strength from eating liver.

But how sure can you be that the animal was healthy at the time of butchering? If the cattle was diseased in any way, that defect was likely to be resident in the liver which contained so large an amount of blood. Therefore, the consumption of liver can be fraught with danger. *If* you prefer iron-rich and protein-rich animal food to vegetable food; and *if* you are sure the liver you consume is from an animal free of taint; and *if* you do not mind ingesting some adrenalin, then perhaps liver would be as good for you as nuts and raisins and avocados, let's say.

The matter of adrenalin caused the eyes of both Dr. Lu and the girl to fly open. I presented the case fairly to them, I believe. "When you are frightened and your muscles suddenly tense in readiness for flight," I explained, "there's been a large squirt of adrenalin into your muscles. That's the big-charge powerhouse *natural* drug that makes your hair stand on end. It's what goes on whenever you are in danger. Well," I appealed to them, "don't you think that the animal in the butchering ramp, ready for slaughter, knows somehow, in some way, that death is about to descend—and that it is frightened? If so, that animal's blood is full of adrenalin. That liver contains about a third of the animal's adrenalin-rich blood. In eating the liver, then, wouldn't you likely be consuming the adrenalin also?"

My listeners made a wry face. I think the butchers had lost customers for their liver right there. Dr. Lu hadn't forgotten about my promise to give my views, as a non-drugging, "anti-shot" doctor, about acupuncture. Like hysterectomies and tonsillectomies and gall bladder removals or appendix removals, it was a current fad. So we turned our eye to the proper end of the telescope and took a look at the *natural* side of things.

THE ENTIRE UNVARNISHED STORY OF ACUPUNCTURE

"I've already given my straight-out, entirely negative opinion of heart surgery," I began, "so maybe I'd better go light on this new acupuncture fad."

"Fad?" Dr. Lu said, a bit sorrowfully. "It's nothing more to you, then? My country's great contribution."

"Sorry, James. But how do we deal here with truth—truth as I know it? Shall I spare anyone's feelings? Or shall I get into the meaty middle of it with pointers that pour light on the thing? Light rather than heat, James—or is this a visceral thing with you because acupuncture is of Chinese origin?"

He smiled apologetically. He was, after all, a man trained to view things with objectivity.

"First, then, James," I said, "I'm against anything and everything, *on a physiological basis,* that uses the human skin as a pincushion. Secondly, I know as a researcher in the natural approaches to healing the sick body, that there is no magic. No special drug or shot or button that'll put health into sick bodies. To get well, one must follow a program. You know the program I mean. Counter-gravitational techniques to make up for the ills of living against gravity, and all the rest.

"Now, you Chinese," I smiled, "you may have given us the wheel and gunpowder and other head-starts toward civilization. But you Chinese, forgive me, have never been known as a nation of supermen in the health department. Acupuncture is widely lauded as the ancient Chinese method of getting people well. The great pain-control method, other apologists call it. But since it has been used and perfected in China for an alleged four thousand years, James, nobody in China ought to be lacking in health. The fact is, however, that you Chinese are at least as sick as the rest of us. So I must view acupuncture as a new gold-producing method rather than an old health-producing one."

"All this reminds me of people who go to seek out a guru and absorb in India the "ancient wisdom of the East." But if India really had all that supercharged brainpower quoted in the saying, "India's ancient wisdom," it appears to me that India would have amounted to much more than it does among the family of nations. A fine nation it probably is, I grant. But if so highly gifted with special wisdom, then why hasn't that wisdom made the place sparkle more than it does on the world scene?

Are the Claims of Acupuncture People True?

"Seems to me that you just can't go repeating something as gospel truth simply because people say it is. There are points to remember. Scientific points. Here they are," and I went on relating my rundown of arguments against acupuncture.

1. The body is not a pincushion.
2. The Chinese are not outstandingly healthy despite the purported wonders of acupuncture.
3. Neurologically, there *are not,* as acupuncturists claim, any "14 meridians of the body" through which flow the forces yin and yang, or anything demonstrable like that.
4. Contrariwise, there *are* nerve centers in the body (ganglia, plexuses, etc.) where the nerve lines can be broken or interrupted. If a needle as long as eight inches is inserted within a human nerve center it can, especially if it is twirled, cause scar-tissue damage and *permanently damage the message-carrying capacity* of nerve pathways. Then the *protective* pain messages cannot get through. It's like taking salicylates (aspirin, anacin) to deaden the ability to react to pain; the trouble goes on unabated but your protective warning signal has been stilled. Of course acupuncture can kill pain. If done improperly it can also multiply pains and permanize pains—a matter hardly ever mentioned. But does the stilling of pain cure anything? Does it make the ailing body well again?

"Sorry, but acupuncture cannot get an OK from any doctor who knows, understands, and deals in *natural* health."

Acupuncture bespeaks the poverty of known healing methods. The fact that so many doctors, money-hungry or plain curious, are making so large a splash about it, indicates how little they have in their own get-well methods. I think that acupuncture is a showy technique that bedazzles people with its dramatics—not unlike that of heart surgery—but is not in any serious sense a get-well program for sick people.

The spectacle of so many old-school doctors on the jump and hustle to use this heroic new little gambit spells out one cogent truth to me. They don't know any real workable method or healing program, so they jump at chimeras and tinsel-rich dramatics. They have entirely missed in their training the health-restoring value of counter-gravitational techniques; of correcting nerve pressures so that functional energy might flow again to sick, deprived organs; of oxygenating the body and purifying the bloodstream and detoxifying the system.

Acupuncture is assuredly an old method. Because of non-performance in really helping the sick get well, it has been side-stepped and gone unused. Now it is being revived. But why?

I think the hustle behind it among so many doctors tells its own story. Acupuncture is an old *nothing-method* with new gold-dust paint on it.

CHAPTER SEVEN

How to Tune Up Your Love Life in Rejuvenating Your Health

This is what will be known a few centuries hence as the Age of Permissiveness. Everybody's excited about sex. And seeing it portrayed, and hearing it discussed, and being aware of it as never before. But still it remains a subject mostly unknown. In spite of all the permissiveness, sex remains a subject that is more talked about and less understood than any other human subject on earth.

This chapter has the intention of changing that general ignorance as far as you are concerned. Here we intend to deal with just about everything you should know about the right and wrong of it, the moral and so-called immoral, the "sex-stuff" you ought to worry about and what you ought to forget.

Is sex necessary? How much of it is necessary? Is there any age when it is not a good and useful factor that tends toward health? Let's present the actual scientific truth—not pseudo-scientific hogwash—about this former hush-hush subject.

Things you ought to know, because they're true.

Things you ought to forget, because they're not true.

The dependable basics about mating, about obtaining healthy orgasms even when mis-mated, about continuing to be sexually nourished even when you do not have a mate at all.

Ready? Let us lift the cover and open the curtains.

IS SEX NECESSARY?

The answer to that one is Yes! And by sex we mean sex that ends in orgasm (or climax). The question should really be: Is it necessary always to finish sexual activity with an orgasm? And the answer is a resounding Yes!

This has to be explained. It needs so straight an explanation that every reader will know once and for all what's behind this pleasant gambit that we call sex.

In the widely, and justifiably, acclaimed Masters-Johnson studies of *Human Sexual Response,** we learned some gutter wisdom. We learned this from what might be called a "gutter woman" or lady of the evening—a prostitute. This poor defrauded female rented out her body to many clients and consented to be examined between clients. In her business, it was known, reaching a climax with a customer was a faked rather then actual thing. Thus she went through the motions of sex without reaching orgasm. (We use the words climax and orgasm interchangeably here; they mean the same.)

Upon examination it was found that her pelvic and genital tissues were engorged with blood. The blood engorgement brought on a state of irritation; this in turn produced inflammation. All this happened after having sex with a customer: sex without climax. With each new sexual encounter the engorgement rose and her pelvic tissues got worse. After the examinations between customers revealed this mounting abnormal state, she was advised to have a climax. It was at the end of her "normal working day" when she'd had sex with several dozen men.

The climax was self-induced by manipulation of the clitoris with her finger. Right after her climax the prostitute was examined again and the swollen pelvic tissues were found to be subsiding. The abnormal blood engorgement was leaving; in a little while it was gone. It proved that sexual activity without reaching orgasm was bad for her. And it proved that sex ending with orgasm was a healthy rather than harmful experience. Why? What makes this so? To clarify the mystery of this—which is almost an everyday matter in our lives and ought to be understood by us—I'd better tell you about a youngish school teacher patient.

HOW MASTURBATION HELPED THIS UPTIGHT FEMALE TEACHER

Miss Bess was a whiz-kid of 25 who'd had her master's degree in education at 22 and was an admittedly talented high school math

---

*Little, Brown & Company, Boston, 1966.

teacher. But despite an outward show of sophisticated insouciance, she revealed in private that she was a mass of inner conflicts—uptight, strained, full of hang-ups. Blessed with a beautiful little figure she was at the same time muddy-colored in complexion, had a bit of unsightly acne at the corner of one jaw, had an everlasting battle with constipation, and walked with a kind of shuffle or slouch instead of squaring back her shoulders to show off her nice bosom.

We have all heard that a person who diagnoses himself or herself has a fool for a patient. Well, Miss Bess had read too many books, believed too much of the self-diagnosing flapdoodle and had a host of labels stuck onto her secret state of conflict.

"I silently adored my father," she confessed to me. "Father-image, I guess. And a lot of 'Momism' too; she was always over-directing me. Then that church we were made to go to—with all the insufferable restrictions they imposed! When I went on my own I got into group therapy and encounters. A bunch of touch sessions and consciousness-raising and some love-ins. But," she murmured half-apologetically, "I'm still a virgin." She felt deeply sorry for herself.

On examination, there was little of a physical nature the matter with her. At the very top of the neck she bore a rather bad nerve pressure, and although this out-of-place atlas vertebra could cause spinal cord pressure and create all kind of havoc in the body below, it was easily corrected. All I needed to do was show her the Head-Lift and the Head-Hang (see *Glossary*) to make sure she continued free of nerve pressure, and that was attended to. Then the Primordial Walk to energize her; the Dowager's Hump to overcome her slouch by straightening her spine; the Knee-Chest resting position to overcome the effects of gravity; plus Diaphragmatic Breathing to reoxygenate her system; and she began to sparkle.

Our little school teacher was given a six-day digestive overhaul—three days of physiological rest by fasting and three days of monodiet eating—and her bowels began to do well. Her muddy color cleared. The acne faded. Her chest came up and she walked with a kind of rhythmic bounce. But the hang-ups and inner conflicts were still there.

I re-examined her. Had I missed anything in her nervous distributions? Was there anything I was not doing that needed doing, or something I was doing that had better be left undone? Not one thing. So I gathered together a little courage and led her into the matter of sex.

"You mentioned being a virgin, young lady. Do you mind being one?"

"Mind? Of course, Doctor. I hate being one and feel the need of *not* being one. But . . . Well, it's fear, I suppose."

I explained the need of regular orgasms as part of a balanced, healthy life and asked if she indulged in sexual reveries. Quite specifically, did she imagine sexual experiences with men she secretly admired?

"Nearly all the time and all the men you can think of," she blurted out with disarming frankness. "I'm forever having the fantasy of being chased by flocks of men, and then being fulfillingly raped by a couple of the handsomer ones. Never fewer than two. Simultaneously!"

Well! That nearly rocked me. I told her about Robie's great work on *Rational Sex*, but she was way ahead of me. I endeavored to introduce her to Krafft-Ebing, Moll, Stekel, Havelock Ellis, but she had read them all. Nevertheless, she was still sexually naive and had never even masturbated in a fulfilling, satisfying way. Momism, oldtime churchly fear of hellfire and brimstone, or whatever it was that could be blamed, there she was needing help.

"Look, I'd just plain out advise you to masturbate," I told her. "Good clitoral stimulation until you achieve good clitoral orgasm." She already knew that the insistence by Freud (and Menninger, Bergler, etc.) on women's having a vaginal orgasm in addition to a clitoral one "as a sign of maturity in the female" had been proved to be so much halfbaked nonsense. She was aware of the value of orgasms, but only in an academic way. She swore earnestly that outside of "feeling delicious" when a hot shower spray fell upon the clitoris or when she combed the pubic hair above it and relished the sensation, she had never in her life completely masturbated.

It was not within my purview of interest to make a value judgment relating to the honesty of her confession. But it was within my province to advise her how best to achieve health. So I really went into the mechanics and techniques of masturbation and instructed her to accomplish full orgasm at least once a week. Then, I promised, as time went along and as the office schedule permitted, I would go into complete details in neurology and physiology that backgrounded my unusual advice. Meanwhile, it was not for her to reason why but just to do it.

Which she did. Really overdid. Being Miss Bess, a confirmed over-achiever, I might have expected it. And just this addition to her program, masturbation on a regular basis, made her completely and thoroughly and wonderfully well. There were reasons for it. Reasons that will give the reader a firm sex background for all the rest of his days. So I'd better spell them out here and now.

WHAT GOES ON DOWN THERE WHEN
YOU'RE SEXUALLY AROUSED?

When the human male is aroused sexually, about eight ounces of blood flow into his sexual organs. This creates the phenomenon of erection. Tissue that is otherwise soft as flesh becomes almost as hard as bone. The erectile tissue of the penis remains thus engorged with blood until he has an orgasm. Then the blood is returned to the circulation, the tension is relieved, the male is bathed in a soothing, relaxed state.

The female pelvis contains about twice as many organs as we find in the male pelvis. Even when not sexually aroused and filled with additional blood, the female pelvis is a crowded place. In about the same space-area as the male pelvis, although shaped a bit differently for birth-giving purposes, the female pelvis contains organs the male has no use for. The ovaries, the uterus, the Fallopian tubes, the broad and round and suspensory ligaments, and so forth, including the urinary bladder, which both sexes have in common. The only organ in that whole pelvic space that the male has and the woman doesn't have is the prostate gland, a tiny thing about the size of a horse chestnut.

Now, what happens when the female gets aroused sexually? In her case about 30 or 32 ounces of blood flow into the genitals. Remember that the woman's pelvis is already a crowded place because of its being laden with a lot of organs. Now add this great amount of blood when she's sexually heated and you have a super-congested mass of organs to deal with. But it's not at all bad *if* she comes to climax. If her mate knows enough to bring her to an orgasm, she's immediately relieved. After her climactic pitch, all that blood begins to seep back into the circulation. With the release of pent-up nervous tension that is the high plateau of the orgasm, the congestion leaves and she, too, is bathed in a pleasant euphoric state.

The brutal fact that we have to face here is that many women do not reach orgasm. Their mates may not know that the women are slower in reaching orgasm and must be treated accordingly in long sexual foreplay. Or the men are interested in their own satisfaction exclusively, and thus do not care about whether the female achieves or does not achieve orgasm. Or the male may be out of control and ejaculate prematurely—with no time or ability thereafter to keep going until the woman reaches a climax.

What's serious is that when there is no climax in the female, that big inflow of 30 ounces of blood is not discharged in any orgastic release of pent-up tension. Instead of flowing back into the circulation it remains there to engorge the female organs. The woman has not been sexually satisfied. She lies awake, tense and nervous, taut as a violin string, waiting for that mass of blood that's congesting her pelvic organs to flow back ever so slowly into her circulation.

When we recall that the female pelvis is a crowded place even without that extra inflow of blood, we come to the great kernel of truth in this whole business. Prolonged congestion produces irritation. Irritation produces inflammation. Inflamed sexual structures represent, in the main, the chief cause of what we call "women's diseases." If there were no inflammations within the female pelvis, I believe there would be no need for that whole speciality known as gynecology.

WHY ARE MEN FASTER IN SEX THAN WOMEN?

I am not sure whether it's worthwhile going into the reasons why men are almost always faster in the sex act than women. Suffice it to say that it's so; it's a neurological effect. The reflex sexual arc to and from the genitals is much longer in the female and shorter in the male—the actual *distance* to travel is shorter in the male, would you believe it? The male appetite for the female can start in the lower pelvis or spinal cord, go from there to his testicles (which produce semen) and penis, then back to the point of origin in the spinal cord. His head does not absolutely have to take part in the business at all.

This explains why prostitution can flourish. A man can walk along with his wife, whom he absolutely adores, and see a hip-swinging wench on the other side of the street, and get a desire to have sex with her right *now*. She may be someone he would never consort with otherwise. A woman beneath him socially, a woman lacking in manners or education or even cleanliness. Yet he's ready to go with her sexually; that is, his pelvis is ready. His interest started in the pelvis and went back to the lower spinal cord in a very short neurological arc. His head didn't have to participate in it very much at all. That's why very fine and high-minded men can at times consort with prostitutes of even the lowest grade.

The woman's sexual interest, however, begins in the brain. Her head has to participate. She has to like or cherish or treasure something about the man first: his voice, musical ability, success, talent, manners. Then this interest seeps down to her pelvis and she becomes sexually aroused. The sexual arc is not from pelvis to pelvis as in the male. It's from head to pelvis and back to the head. This is why the female adores kissing and petting after the orgasm (back to the head), while the male says that after his orgasm he's had the main course and doesn't care to go back to the appetizer.

So there's a large part of the answer to why men are faster in the sex act than women. His sexual interest may start and end in the pelvis; but hers must begin in the head. Therefore, the unknowing man—not knowledgeable about women and their parts and patterns—quickly reaches his climax, feels satisfied and fine, turns over and goes to sleep in blissful relaxation. And the woman who has this person for a mate—she cannot relax for hours, or until all that blood flows slowly back in the circulation, the blood that would have been disgorged at once if she'd had her climax. If her mate had known! Had he been knowledgeable about women!

WHAT MUST A MAN KNOW ABOUT WOMEN'S PARTS?

So what would a man need to know to make him knowledgeable in this frame of reference? He would have to know about the female erogenous zones—the parts that most quickly arouse her. That's one thing. And it would be useful to know how to use a few skills to make those zones blossom into peak performance.

First, in general, it's useful to know that men and women are not really worlds apart. Before his birth, while still a fetus in his mother's womb, he might have come out a girl as easily as a boy. What are now his testicles would have remained upstairs and been ovaries. The scrotum, or sac which contains the testicles, would have composed the lips of the vagina. Even his penis would have remained in the very same spot and been a clitoris—really a very tiny penis in the female with some of the same functions. And, he ought to know, the reason why his breast nipples are sexually excitable is that he has a rudimentary milk-factory setup there not too unlike that of the female's.

The lips are of course erogenous zones. The man ought to fondle and kiss his mate long before he permits himself to become sexually aroused. Once he becomes sexually excited, he may come to the point of no return much sooner than he'd like. When he has stimulated the woman enough to get her interested and ready, the lips he's kissing will swell and turn suddenly warmer. And—note well!—the insides of the lips will become very hot indeed and very moist also.

The nipples of the breasts, and the tissue right around them, are sex-arousing zones. They ought to be stroked, fondled, kissed, nibbled—anything that will be exciting. When the nipples become hard, that's another sign the woman is on the way to true arousal. In the four phases of the human sexual response that is what is called the excitement phase; Phase No. 1. The lubricating fluid starts flowing and the vagina becomes moist. Even erotic thoughts alone will bring on this excitement phase, but a man's direct contact with her genitals will make the woman respond much quicker.

In the male, the penis becomes engorged with blood during this phase and a small penis will double in size. Inside the vagina there is a "sweating action" centered in the walls of the vestibule. The large outer lips of the vagina will widen with blood engorgement and expose the two inner lips. The circular sphincter muscles of the vagina, like hoops around a barrel, will become tense. The vagina (barrel) itself undergoes an interesting change. The first third tenses, as though to grip the penis tightly, while the remaining two-thirds elongates about an inch and balloons to something like three times its usual size.

THE SIZE OF THE PENIS MAKES NO DIFFERENCE

This ought to settle for all time the matter that bothers so many men who believe themselves "under-endowed" in penis size. Women are every bit as sexually thrilled and satisfied with small men as with big men, since only the first third of the vagina can really grip the male organ. The determinant is whether the woman likes the man or loves him. If she is enraptured with his personality or other qualities, the size of the penis makes no difference. It's only when they talk or joke aimlessly that women refer to the supposed value of the large penis. In actuality, many women have confided, a small man who is dear to them is far more attractive and desirable than a "large-built" man who isn't.

The talk that one hears is to the effect that Negro men are especially large-built or well endowed in this respect. The truth is that the black man's penis is usually longer in the relaxed state, but not in any important respect larger than the white man's penis in the erect state. No one seems to know why this is so. It just happens that when a white man has an erection his penis enlarges much more from the "soft stage" than is the case with the average black man. This has been observed by many researchers.

As to the length of the penis, that too is unimportant. The reason for this is that the nerve supply from the walls of the vagina is really present only in the front part of the vagina. Toward the inner or back portion, the vagina has virtually no feeling. Thus all that fiction about the long penis being able to hit the cervix (neck of the womb) and provide extra excitement is ready to be discarded also.

THE FEMALE HAS A "LITTLE PENIS" ALSO

The female clitoris may properly be called a little penis. It, also, is fitted with a "head" and a foreskin. It contains the same kind of erectile tissue as the male organ. It gets hard when sexually excited. The prepuce (foreskin) can become hooded or over-hooded and need to be circumsized—and at times this can relieve a certain type of frigidity. Most of all, the head of the clitoris, like the head of the male penis, is the chief zone of the libido. It is the head and front of sexual arousal.

It is the clitoris that should be stimulated in the petting, kissing and general foreplay of sex. This makes the woman ready for sex activity and heads her toward achieving an orgasm. Over the years women have complained to me in the office that they do not get sufficient sexual pleasure because their husbands "ride low." By this they meant that in the conventional male-superior position of sex, the male position was too low to contact and stimulate the clitoris during the in-and-out movements of the act.

These women were not on the right track. (I always thought that they didn't much like their mates anyway; for if they did, his "ride low" position would have been thoroughly satisfactory.) Here are the facts. Even if the man is much shorter than his wife, or if he prefers to lie over her with his face below hers rather than above her head, her clitoris will be stimulated. Of course it is better if the positioning is such that with every movement the man's pubic hair and pubic bone hit the clitoris and stimulate it. But no matter what the male position is, the clitoris gets worked on. The inner lips of the vagina undergo a pull-and-release motion as the in-and-out movement of the penis proceeds. Being pulled and released by the inserting and retracting motion of the penis, these inner lips pull on the clitoris to which they are attached above. The inner lips (labia minora) converge above, or toward the front, at the clitoris. It is impossible for the man to go through the in-and-out inserting and retracting of his organ without causing the clitoris to get pulled and released in the process.

Thus the clitoris gets a workout, no matter what. The big question is whether it gets a workout *long* enough, and *early* enough before the man has his orgasm and quits his movements, for the woman to mount to orgastic heights.

SEE THAT PUBIC HAIRS TOUCH:
HAIR CONDUCTS ELECTRICITY

We come to the biggest mystery question of all: What *is* sex? Volumes have been written about this, but the answers have never been entirely, all-embracingly satisfactory. One cannot be at doctoring for more than four decades, as I have, and not come up with an answer or theory about sex—he can't, unless it is a mere moneymaking business instead of a dedication. So here is my thinking about the why and how of sex.

The nearest we can define it is that sex is an electro-magnetic interchange between the male and female. The male represents the electric; the female is the magnetic. The magnet attracts—and females certainly attract males. The electric lunges out and seeks, hunting its ground area—and the male certainly hunts and seeks the female as the place where he wants to *be grounded.*

In straight logic one would expect the woman to chase the man, rather than the way it is. That would be logical because it is the man that expends in sex. He gives up his strength in it. Out of his loins flow the most vital mineral salts and precious fluids of the body—so vital and precious that they can make another body and form another life. That's what happens when the man ejaculates in sex. So he loses something. But the woman gains in sex. Her vaginal walls absorb the male's precious fluids; if there is anything like love in the union she is energized and profited by the act, losing nothing out of her store of vital fluids. So why does the male chase the female rather than the other way around? Why—unless it is that the act is an electro-magnetic interchange and the magnet attracts just as the steel magnet attracts metal to itself.

Human hair is a great conductor of electricity. This includes pubic hair, of course. Human beings alone seem to have pubic hair, and only human beings seem to have sex (conventionally at least) in the chest-to-chest postion. In this position the *pubic hairs of male and female are in contact.* We know how the hair makes electric sparks when we run a comb through it. When the pubic hair of lovers is in contact, with ensuing friction, the electric sparks fly also. It lends toward the electro-magnetic interchange I speak of. This is my own theory of sex. I think it holds up as well as any other I have ever encountered.

HARDLY ANYTHING THAT YOU DO IN BED CAN BE WRONG

Mrs. Grant, a woman well into middle age, was interested in my telling her that only the first third of the vagina can really *feel*. She hated the whole business of sex, she said, because her husband "made her" do things she didn't like. What things? She made a wry face.

"It's awful to have to satisfy him orally." Her hands went up in horror. "Doctor Morrision, it's a nasty perversion!"

"Don't label things," I said sternly.

She was in need of semantic truths in place of her semantic misdirections. I explained the difference between perversion and perversity. If a person needs to act out some out-of-the-usual sexual position or fetish, it's a perversion only if he or she can get no sexual gratification at all without this unusual act. If it is a once-in-a-while act, something like a fun thing or as an occasional stimulus to sex, it is merely a perversity. The person is perverse—not perverted. Prisoners confined to their own sex sometimes perform homosexual acts. Yet this is a perversity instead of a perversion *in those circumstances.* Once free and able to consort with the opposite sex, these people prefer heterosexual experiences. Thus, even homosexual activity—as a temporary thing—is not a perversion. "So don't be quick to label people," I warned.

She saw I was rather provoked with her and insisted on talking about the matter. During the conversation I got to the real nubbin of it. She had read Kinsey and others and knew that oral sex, or fellatio in this case, was not at all unusual. The truth was that she had read about men satisfying women orally and desired to experience this herself, but was afraid to ask. "It's my hang-up." she said. "It's got so that I imagine myself with all kinds of beautiful men people, all of them doing that to me. And I've developed a deep guilt-feeling about it. My upbringing sets off that guilty sense, I guess."

I told her then that she ought to keep a sign hanging in her bedroom, as one writer suggested. The sign should read: *Nothing that you can do in bed is wrong.* I would amend that only slightly, for while I believe that hardly anything between consenting adults can be wrong, inflicting pain, as in sado-masochistic (S/M) acts, or even profound bondage-degradation (B/D) in the name of sex, can be traumatic and harmful.

"As to your upbringing," I declared, "my hope is that soon all churches will humanize sex standards and not be so righteously uptight about sex practices. Possibly the most baneful influence on your life is that puritanical 'good solid upbringing' of yours—one whose rigid dogmatisms ought to be neutralized out of you. If yours, in the department of sex, was a good upbringing," I insisted, "what you need now is a good downbringing. Down to realities."

EVERYBODY HAS SEXUAL HANG-UPS

She had mentioned her hang-up on desiring oral sex. Since this triggered in her a deep guilt-sense, I told her something she very much needed to know. The truth. The matter of coming to grips with realities in this area. All people I'd ever known had some kind of sex hang-ups. Imaginings and reveries and fantasies of one kind or another. Her eyes fairly popped as I recited the ones that had come to my attention during 40 years.

Some people cannot enjoy sex unless they imagine themselves having it with a person of another race or color. Some men can get excited only when visualizing breasts of enormous size—and some women must phantasize themselves being entered by a very large male organ. There are people who have hang-ups on hairy bodies, hair*less* bodies, short stocky men built like slabs of marble, long stemmed American beauties whose looks don't count if the legs are long and slim. There are women who can get turned on mostly, or even only, by beanpole-thin men, and men who can get excited only by roly-poly women. Some like their mates to have strong odors emanating from their armpits, skins, genitals; others abhor all body odors, fair or foul. There are even people whose secret hang-up is having sex with one-legged opposites, or cripples of other kinds.

"These are your peers," I declared quite clearly. "I'm talking about your equals, not people out of skid row. Deep inside, most people have hang-ups of some kind. So what? They don't hurt anyone. You are not alone in your special hang-up."

She treasured these words. Her pleased thanks showed genuine relief. The phrase: "These are your peers, your equals," appeared to give her mental tranquility. In a moment she was cured of her guilt sense. Just knowing that others had the same thing, or worse, was what did it.

"So if oral sex is what you desire," I concluded, "just go ahead and suggest it to your husband. He'll probably be tickled that you asked. The lips of the vagina can be made every bit as clean as those of the mouth. And if germs worry you, they can be transferred better in mouth-kissing than in cunnilingus." I paused to make sure this sank in. "So you kids go on and have a ball," I urged.

She needed a bit more assurance. Or perhaps she merely wanted to act out a dramatic urge inside her.

"Can't older people—like us—forget about sex?"

I didn't think that this query was exactly honest. She did not believe herself old, and she did not wish to forget sex. Was she posing or acting out a virtue she wanted me to believe she had?

"No," I said in clipped accents. "What you don't use, you lose. Older people need sex also. Even antediluvian people in your age bracket," I couldn't help adding.

She backed down and asked, a little timorously, if "it was all right to try different positions in sex, too?" This recalled to mind the extraordinary experience I had with Nan, a fortyish woman who was quite a character.

HINTS ON REJUVENATING SEXUAL CAPABILITIES

This lady said that she had heard me declare something quite startling in a lecture she had attended. I'd said that if you took a sunbath on the spleen, it could give you more sexual vigor. This was almost, though not quite, what I had said in my lecture, but it was good enough as a starter. What she came to the office about was her husband's impotence. "He can't perform in bed," she said freely and frankly, not at all bashful about it. "It's in his mind, I think. If you knew him, Doctor, you'd know what a creep the guy is."

Well! This was not the kind of conversation I liked. If the woman thought she was impressing me with sophistication, or whatever, she wasn't. Later I was to discover that her husband was not impotent; but that she had a lover who was, and she sought help for him.

What to Do About Impotence

Impotence is an overused word, and a misinterpreted one. In by far the majority of cases it is actually, as Nan indicated, in the mind. Although she meant it disparagingly about her husband (who wasn't impotent at all, it developed later), the truth is that almost always the man's inability "to perform in bed" is not due to his inability to have an erection. The rule is as follows: If a man can have an erection at any time at all, then the erection mechanism is there, the ability is present, and he is not physically incompetent. Nearly all men have what they call "a morning erection." Thus nearly all men have the equipment for erection. Impotence must therefore be due to another cause.

Over the years men have told me their reasons for being unable to perform. Being laughed at or humiliated by women was the reason most often given. At times they had the ill-luck to cohabit with younger women who hurried them, or called them "Grandpa" or otherwise ridiculed them. This hurt their self-esteem and confidence. If a man believes that he might not be able to satisfy his partner in sex, very often he cannot. It has been said—a bit inelegantly but rather graphically—that imagination is as good as a physic for a fool.

Some studies had in fact shown that sexual vigor is increased when one exposed the spleen to the sun for as much as an hour. If this is done before 10 in the morning or after 4 in the afternoon, when your shadow is longer than you are tall, which is the safety rule in sunbathing, then the splenic area right below your left ribs may be sunbathed for an hour while the rest of the body is covered with light gauze or cheesecloth. For reasons not clearly understood, one such exposure for an hour every six months is enough to increase sexual capacity to a noticeably great degree. This was what I had said in a lecture, the one Nan said she had attended. Would her impotent husband be made competent by such a sunbath, she wanted to know.

Nan, however, had other ideas she wished to air. In a brief time, she confessed that her marriage was incompatible and she had a lover who needed all kinds of stimuli to be able to perform sexually. Despite this, she said, she loved him "devotedly" and would do everything possible to help him (or herself).

HOME SEX MOVIES AND APHRODISIACS

"He wants to try not only different positions but home sex movies and aphrodisiac (sex-arousing) foods and the lot," she said. "When and where ought we to stop?" When I indicated that I could not see any valid objection to her trying all the positions she could think of, or even lewd movies if that was what was desired, but would object only to overeating protein foods, for that was what the sex-arousing foods were at bottom, the true purpose of her inquiry came to the surface.

"And spanking? Is that all right too?" she asked.

This shocked me a little. I waited for her to explain, which I knew she was itching to do.

"My—well, my friend, likes to swat me a little. He isn't too rough, understand. And I must confess I like it too. It does something to both of us."

If it was only that, and nothing violent, I assured her that it was only another hang-up. Some had one kind and some another. If no tissues were bruised, I could find no professional reason to prohibit their games; the moral issues, if any, were not in my province. But for the impotence, real or fancied, I had a few suggestions which belonged in my area of interest.

For the low sex interest, as evidenced by the need for so much stimulation by way of pornographic movies and the like, foods rich in iodine have at times been found to upgrade the libido. Thus I could recommend fresh pineapple, raw onions and even frequent meals of salt water fish, freshly caught and lightly broiled. If the counter-gravitational factors were attended to, the iodine-rich foods could be fully appropriated by the system, particularly if the nerves to the digestion organs were at the same time freed of existing pressures. (See *Glossary*.) Also, it seemed wise for the man to take a few spoonfuls of yeast every day for the Vitamin B content, because there appeared to be a relationship between the niacin in yeast and one's low sex drive. For protein intake I suggested meals almost exclusively made up of wheat germ, for over the years I'd discovered that wheat germ was not only just about the best of proteins and the cheapest to buy, but also was a kind of sex invigorator, especially when sweetened with honey. Over and above all this, I advised the so-called impotent man to take 100 I.U. of organic Vitamin E after each meal; all of which did not appear to help very much until he also followed the Missing Link get-well programs relating to counter-gravity and pinched nerves; whereupon Nan reported gleefully that her "friend" now was super-perfect because "he had his sexual trotting harness on at all times."

HOW TO HELP HEAL THE PROSTATE GLAND AT HOME

It doesn't take too many years of practice for a doctor to become aware of a curious characteristic in men. They don't like to talk about their sexual needs and shortcomings. In many cases they send their wives to have the consultation about them *in absentia*. One *gran dama* of the landed Spanish aristocracy, Sra. Guadalupe, was one of these Messengers for the Lord and Master.

"He has big prostrate trouble," she said blushingly.

"You mean prosTATE," I corrected.

"Well, he cannot pass the water for a long time. I mean he must wait for a long time to start. And he burns doing it sometimes."

I have found to my complete satisfaction that an enlarged or inflamed prostate gland is due to three major reasons in our *civilized* society. First, there is always a nerve pressure problem associated with prostatitis. Often the pinched nerve is found in the lower back, but sometimes it may be a referred nerve-pressure interference from as far away as the atlas vertebra at the very top of the neck. I have never seen a single case of prostate trouble without *some* nerve-pinching state accompanying it. This, fortunately, can be corrected in most cases by the nerve-unpinching or *vertebra-adjusting drills* given in Chapter 12, plus the easy counter-gravitational programs that at the same time help many other conditions. (See *Glossary.*)

Second, the reason the prostate gland is subject to disturbing ailments is precisely because we live against gravity. The weight of the body above bears down in never ceasing strain upon the little prostate gland. Even the weight of the urinary bladder just above it exerts a steady gravity-stress on the gland. If we were horizontal animals, with the weight evenly distributed over four points by way of hind legs and forelegs, the prostate would not be constantly bearing the weight-load of everything above it. Moreover, we are today the end-result of all the strains and stresses we have borne in all our lifetime; and some of the falls or twists or jars we've sustained have caused the pelvis to slip downward in front. The chiropractor can fix this by lifting the tendon of Gracilis out of the spasm that this tendon always suffers in prostatitis. Lacking chiropractic attention, or not desiring it, the technique that teaches how to *Abduct Thighs,* plus the Pelvic Back-Tip and the Primordial Walk will in most cases alleviate the condition.

Third—the most sensitive reason of all. It is the tendency of men to *maintain an erection for too long a time.* I am convinced of this after watching cases of prostatitis and inquiring into the habits of those I've treated. The gland manufactures a fluid which must be mixed with semen to thin the semen down—else the seminal fluid would be too "gluey" to flow. When sexually aroused, the little prostate gland is engorged and making its own prostatic fluid. Being a tender organ, it should not be overworked. So long as the man has an erection, it is working. If the male seeks to squeeze out of sex more pleasure than is normal (for a longer time, really), then the prostate gland is working for a longer time than need be. This happens when a man "teases" his sex play too much; holds on to the erection for a very long time, meanwhile overburdening the working time of the prostate gland. Being overtaxed, it becomes inflamed. Being inflamed, it swells to larger and harder size outwardly, and also inwardly. Since the tube through which the male urinates goes through this gland, when it swells inwardly it blocks the free flow of urine.

Admittedly, some prostatic problems have gone too far to be healed by nature; then they need to be repaired by surgery—which is not truly healing, but just repair-work. (The failure of the physician is the opportunity of the surgeon.) But having seen hundreds of cases of prostatitis I can say unequivocally that very few cannot be helped by natural means. The reason so many are referred to surgery is that the surgeons, and the doctors who refer such cases to the surgeons, have not studied natural healing methods which include adjusting the body to a state of mechanical rightness *as a machine* (for no machine that is out of adjustment can be reasonably expected to work properly), and compensating for the counter-gravitational strains and stresses, and reoxygenating the system, and giving it a physiological rest which also purifies the bloodstream—the Missing Link programs, in short, that are here offered. (See *Glossary*.) Not being trained in these techniques, these doctors and surgeons cannot of course do them or recommend them. Thus they do what they *can* do: surgical repair.

A note of importance. When any doctor says that "everything possible is being done" you must ask yourself whether it is true. Usually this is said when a case is failing and the family shows concern or displeasure. So when the doctor says, in defense, that "everything possible is being done," to indicate that they have left no stone unturned, ask him (or yourself) this simple self-protective question. Are they really doing everything? Or merely everything within their own system of healing, within the close boundaries of their special healing approach? Everything, etymologically, would mean *all things*. It would mean that they are using methods of doctors trained differently from the way they've been trained. Everything to help, to save a life.

In addition to the Missing Link programs set forth in the *Glossary* of this book, there are some specific items of help for the man with an enlarged prostate. Enlarged, hard, inflamed—all of this happens to the gland.

Sitting on a hot water bottle has been found to be a quite useful means of self-help. I used to instruct the wife to have a hot water bottle filled and waiting on the seat used by her husband, meaning the chair which he occupied during the dinner hour. If too hot to be borne, a towel is folded over it. He sits atop the rubber bottle with confidence, for his body weight will not cause it to burst. There is a kind of emanation akin to infra-red heat radiation, and this travels upward as his weight presses down on the bottle, and is absorbed by his nether body. The prostate tends to soften under this treatment. Merely an hour or so spent while at the dinner table, and results are often most satisfactory.

Sometimes a cold sitz bath is unexpectedly effective. This is done at night, when the patient will not go out anymore for the day (and risk taking cold). He lowers himself into a basin that will accommodate his body only up to his lower spine in back and the pelvis in front. Thus the concentration is on his middle, where the prostate is located, instead of being dispersed over the entire body. When once accustomed to the cold, ice cubes should be added. Fifteen minutes in this kind of sitz bath can reduce an inflamed, very enlarged gland to where urination is easy again.

Diaphragmatic breathing, as described in the *Glossary,* should most especially be done in prostatic difficulty. Organic Vitamin E, 200 to 400 International Units, is helpful in many cases when taken after meals, preferably after the fatty meal of the day. Sexual activity should be limited to "doing it and getting it done" instead of stretching it out, with injury to the overworked gland.

CONDOMS ARE NON-CONDUCTORS OF MALE ELECTRICITY

Bruce and Connie were married barely a year and already the young man had nagging back pains that he'd never had before. She, it appeared, had insisted on their using contraceptive methods; and since neither knew much about it they settled on using condoms because it was the easiest choice. Connie was irregular in her menstrual periods and worried each month lest the condoms hadn't worked.

Of all the ways to prevent conception, the condom has least to recommend it in my opinion. You will remember that sex, if we understand anything about it at all, is an electro-magnetic interchange. During the sex act, the male is exchanging his electric thrusts while absorbing the female magnetic emanations. *But rubber is a nonconductor of electricity;* and the rubber condom is guilty of preventing the healthy conduction, or flow, of the male electrical discharges. The current is halted by the non-conductor. The neurological arc is not completed; it is thwarted. It can cause severe backaches in even young and very strong newly-married men who never used condoms before. I have seen this in practice too many times to doubt my theory. Moreover, when I halt the use of condoms the backaches go away, which is confirmatory evidence of the theory.

WHY "THE PILL" IS HARMFUL

What about the other forms of preventing conception? First, we must set down what is important about "The Pill" because it is being so widely touted and used these days. I would not permit a loved one of mine to use "The Pill." I base this on the very best of physiological reasons. The human female body is composed of several trillion cells—all of them put together to express that "mother hunger" which is the peg on which the onward march of civilization swings. *Preservation of the species*—that's what the built-in female "mother hunger" guarantees. And anything which can thwart this great built-in physiological hunger must be harmful to the organism. To advise a woman to take "The Pill" is to deal with imponderables at her expense. It'll take several decades before we know the end-result of monkeying with natural human urges in this way. It ought not be recommended to unknowing, innocent young people who have confidence in the doctor's "knowingness." If the pressures from the anxious-to-sell drug firms were not so insistently great on the doctors, perhaps the latter would not jump on "The Pill" bandwagon so indiscriminately—and we'd not see so many uterine hemorrhages and suchlike resulting from "The Pill."

WHAT'S GOOD AND BAD ABOUT
THE OTHER CONTRACEPTIVES

The *intra-uterine device* (IUD) is currently popular. There is not yet sufficient evidence against it, but again, on the basis of physiology, it is probably a wrong device to use. I have a close friend who owns a five-story hospital in Mexico City, one with over a hundred rooms housing many assorted patients. He has himself done more than 14,000 surgical operations and is a careful student of human ills. Just prior to this writing, he informed me (in a discussion of this subject) that he has found evidence of cancer in the Fallopian tubes which he attributes to the back-up influence of the intra-uterine device. These cancerous degenerations he observed not in one but in a succession of those who wore the IUD. My friend's opinion, though not at all conclusive, is enough to warrant my advising young people to stay away from the IUD, even the new one with release setups, especially when there are other contraceptive methods without horrendous possibilities.

Vasectomy is usually a dependable contraceptive method if the man is very sure that he will never again want children. There is some talk about one's being able to untie the blockage and make propagation possible again, but this is not dependably true. *Withdrawal* (coitus interruptus) is highly unsatisfactory for several reasons. It can be a nerve-shattering practice always to keep in mind withdrawing at the peak moment of pleasure. As in the case of the condom, it can "burn out" the insulation that protects the nerve lines active in the electro-magnetic interchange of sex—and often causes backaches by reason of thwarting the natural sexual expression. Worst of all, it is not very safe or dependable. Long before the actual ejaculation, there are several drops of semen-laden fluid at the end of the penis. These are formed during the male's "warm-up arousal period" much as two similar glands in the female genitalia form a lubricating fluid in her—and these fluid droplets can impregnate the woman.

Douching is fine for cleanliness but can be a lost cause in contraception. It is true that a spoonful of vinegar in about two quarts of water will destroy the male sperm. But will it do that soon enough? The answer is a conclusive negative. It cannot ever be depended upon to do this. The *Rhythm Method* is similarly undependable, although it does have a reasonable basis in physiology. The trouble is that one's menstrual rhythm can change without warning. It is virtually impossible to set up one's exact ovulation times by the calendar. *Abstinence*—if one can really abstain from sex—can be recommended as a great builder of character and disciplinary strength. But in the long run I do not think it is good for one's health. The rule in physiology is: what you do not use, you lose. Nature takes away those functions which you do not employ. Unless abstinence is a matter of deep religious conviction. I would advise against it.

Dismissing both the pessary and suppository as inefficient and undependable, this leaves only *the diaphragm* for serious consideration. I believe that a well-fitted diaphragm is the best contraceptive device yet invented. The advantages are many. The woman does not know that she is wearing anything at all, provided always that it was properly and carefully fitted—not done in a rush-rush doctor's office where the idea was to assembly-line the patient out of the way to make room for next and next-next. The man is entirely unaware that any device has been interposed to stop his sperm from entering the cervical opening. Unlike the condom, which halts conduction of electro-magnetic forces in sex, here the rubber is only at the end of the vaginal vestibule and the walls of the vagina are free to absorb both the male seminal deposits and electrical emanations.

To make assurance doubly sure, I recommend that even with the best fitted diaphragm one ought to be re-fitted every two years. The size of the vaginal vault may alter imperceptibly. Unwanted pregnancies, in my experience, have occurred among users of the diaphragm only when new fittings have not been attended to or new and relatively fresh diaphragms were allowed to dry out during non-use.

HOW TO STRENGTHEN THE SEX MUSCLES
AND OTHER AIDS

An easy and effective way to strengthen the vaginal muscles involved in gripping the penis is this. Imagine your needing to evacuate the bowels and *draw back the stool forcefully*. You cannot do this without working the sphincters and strengthening them. Another way to build strength into the muscles of the vagina is to place a large coin between the buttocks and walk around gripping the coin between the "cheeks of the posterior." Still another sex-muscle strengthener is that of sitting on the floor flat on the buttocks and then "walking with your buttocks as legs." This means that you propel yourself with one buttock for one step, then the opposite buttock propels you one step further, and so on. Your legs do not help in the operation. You actually move forward by having the buttocks do all the work of *walking* you.

Men can also stengthen the muscles involved in sex. In their case, the most direct exercise is that of consciously pulling back the urine. Imagine your needing to urinate and having no handy place for it. This would call for your *holding back;* for pulling it inward. This exercises and strengthens the coccygeus muscles involved. Another way to strengthen the involved muscles is to stand and think—concentrate hard—about raising and extending the penis. After a few attempts, this will actually happen. Your concentrating on this will cause you to apply power in the right area, and you will see the penis moving forward and upward. If this is done with regularity, the strength is built into the organ, and then you can extend and lift the penis *at will* when it is inside the vagina.

For some degree of protection against infection, the male can rub a little vinegar onto the glans, or head, of his penis. The acid of vinegar is sufficient to destroy most VD microorganisms *if* contacted in time. This does not constitute sure protection by any means. Nonetheless, when several men consorted sexually with infected women, it has been reported that those who had rubbed vinegar into their penis-skin avoided the disease while their mates, not so protected, did not. In this connection, also, it is useful to know the role that alcohol plays in contacting gonorrheal or syphilitic infections. When groups of drinking and non-drinking sailors had sex with the same prostitutes, those with alcohol in their blood were infected, while the non-drinking men had no disease after-effects at all. This has been reported with enough sufficiency to give it credibility. It would appear that the gonococci which are supposed to be the pathogenic or causative germs of gonorrhea, and the spriochete pallida on which syphillis is blamed, do not like people without alcohol in their blood. Being parasites, they seem to enjoy feeding on alcohol-soaked tissue.

Sex Needs for All

This important chapter on the important matter of sex ought to be closed, I think, with this final word. Every adult in the world needs sex—or at least sexual orgasms from time to time. It is a healthy expression of life. For the elderly, sex is, I am convinced, a kind of insurance against premature death. And it does not matter *physiologically* how the orgasms are obtained! In the absence of a sexual partner, I believe the widow or widower can profit by self-induced orgasms—by way of masturbation.

To the human system it does not matter how sex is achieved. The four plateaus of orgasm are exactly the same whether they are reached by erotic thinking, or masturbation or homosexual or heterosexual activity, or any kind of reveries or fantasizing. Physiologically, it is all the same—and of benefit. In the matter of sex with love attached, that is another matter. Then the orgasm is exactly the same *physio*logically, but not the same *psycho*logically. Naturally, when there is an interchange of loving attitudes and responses in addition to the actual physical contact, there is a psychological benefit also. But that is icing on the cake. For sheer physical benefit, be it remembered, any kind of sexual climax is beneficial, however induced.

CHAPTER EIGHT

How to Swiftly Restore Youthful Vigor to Your Legs and Feet

We know that "horizontal" animals have their weight more or less evenly distributed on four feet. "Vertical" human beings, however, bear all the weight of the body upon two small structures, the feet, which, when side by side, occupy but a very tiny area of ground. Yet the entire superstructure—all of the body above those feet—must be borne and balanced by that small area below. It is not architecturally or structurally feasible or correct that the large mass of human body was made to support itself on so small a space.

Any wonder the feet of human beings get into trouble?

Now consider the legs on which we depend for transporting the upper body, and for holding us aloft and upright. Both the legs and feet catch the heavy strains and stresses of living against gravity. Thus we have widespread fallen arches, varicose veins, "trick knees" which just won't behave, painful sciatica cases, and the like. The way those legs and feet of ours bear the brunt of jarring falls and mis-steps and twists and turns, there is ample reason for their troubles so long as we live against gravity—which will be forever, most likely.

But we can do things about it. This chapter will show us how: how to compensate for our straight-up, counter-gravitational style of living; what to do to overcome varicose veins, flat feet, nerve pressures and painful sciatica and similar ills.

HOW TO RAISE FALLEN ARCHES
MOST NATURALLY AND EFFECTIVELY

Did you know that, structurally considered, you are an inverted pyramid? Yes, you most certainly are. From the time you first lifted yourself into upright position from your baby crib, you have been like a pyramid upside down. Broad at the shoulders, tapering down to two small feet; balancing yourself precariously upon that little space taken up by your feet.

Every time you ever jumped in your life, your feet got the sharp whack and jolt of your weight right down smack upon them. The seven bones which comprise the arch are often jarred out of position. When the middle keystone ones of those seven bones drop down, they can pinch the end nerves of a very long nerve pathway from the backbone all the way down the legs. Thus there is often a backwash pain that goes *upward* from the feet to the legs to the lower backbone.

HOW GERALD HANDLED HIS FOOT ARCH PAINS

Gerald Connelly was a high school principal who'd been a patient at the office before my retirement, and we'd become quite friendly. His wife, Dr. Elizabeth, who had also gone to the top as an educator, knew very well our natural approaches to healing, for she was a patient at the office under the care of a young associate. Thus, when Gerald got into deep trouble, she took hold and knew what to do.

Working in his garden, my friend stepped on a jutting stone and suffered profound pain in what is called the transverse arch of the foot. For days he hobbled around, but kept on working. Then his ankle swelled and intolerable pain shot up his leg. The doctors he consulted gave him drugs to still the pain. But he had suffered a badly fallen arch with associated tibial nerve pressure, and this was neither investigated nor treated. At last the pain crept upward into his back and he was completely helpless. All this, mind you, because he needed his flat foot adjusted upward to lift the pressure off that posterior tibial nerve.

Dr. Elizabeth phoned to my retirement home on the opposite coast of the nation and ordered me to stand by—they were flying out. That's the kind of dominant woman she was. Her husband was in agony and I was his friend, retired or not.

Big deal! All I had to do was lift two little bones that go by the fancy name of cuneiforms and the agony disappeared. The bones weren't pinching the nerve anymore; he didn't need pain-killing drugs anymore; he smiled for the first time in weeks.

Now, what I had done he could have done for himself—a bit more slowly but just as effectively. In fact, to continue the treatment, I gave Gerald the technique that would probably have done the job all by itself, without my intervention.

THE SMART WAY TO REBUILD YOUR ARCHES—
USE A ROLLING PIN

The last thing at night, take a foot bath in luke-warm water. This softens the tissues of the feet. Now, get into your pajamas or night dress and be ready to jump into bed without the need for walking around anymore, for whatever reason. At your bedside keep an old-fashioned rolling pin. Holding on to two chair-backs for balance, step onto the rolling pin with *both* feet, even though only one foot may need the treatment. Now roll on that pin, supporting yourself by the furniture to keep from falling. Roll as far front as you can, clear to the toes; then as far back as possible, almost to the heels. Do this back and forth as many times as you can stand the pain, for the foot in need of this arch-lifting technique will be protesting as the rolling motion lifts the flattened arch. Then, when you can stand no more rolling, step off the rolling pin *directly* into bed. *No more walking around to pound down what you had lifted up.*

The foot bath has softened the tissues of the feet. The rolling pin has raised the bones of the arch. For the ensuing eight hours or so you will be off your feet, not pounding the arch down. In a month or six weeks of this technique, applied regularly every night, you can rebuild fallen arches all by yourself. And do the job well, with complete technical correctness. If a rolling pin isn't available, use two cylindrical (not curved) empty bottles.

It happens quite often that severe low-back pain does not quit, regardless of the treatments given you by your chiropractor, because some of the trouble comes from below. In such cases, while your upper body is being put into adjustment at the vertebral column, you can help at the feet with this self-help technique.

HOW TO HANDLE SCIATICA

Speaking of retirement, I must set down the case of the man who decided to zero in on me way down in Guadalajara, Mexico, where I was living and writing in my retirement home. Dr. Roberts, a full professor at a university, had a truly violent siege of sciatica and decided he needed me because I'd helped him out of difficult things years before. The man's sciatic nerve pains were so great that rivulets of perspiration fairly streamed from his forehead when he attempted to stand, much less walk.

A surprising communication reached me in Guadalajara. "What right have you to retire? You're too young anyway. Do you recall putting me to bed for my heart problem with what you fancily called a *complete physiological rest?* I remember one thing: your saying that my heart would save in three days of rest the energy of sixty thousand heartbeats. Well, having saved me once, I'm now your responsibility. I'm plagued with the worst case of sciatica that you or any colleague of yours ever saw."

It was curious how this came about. Dr. Roberts had a mole on the back of his neck that rubbed against his collar. They said it was a serious and very threatening melanoma and he submitted to surgery. In some unaccountable manner, the surgery triggered the recurrence of sciatica that he'd had as a college student some 35 years earlier.

This time the pain all along his leg was more severe than that of years ago. The usual pain-killing drugs did not help. When he arrived he was groggy from sedation. "The pain's rising through the thresh-hold, Doctor," he smiled bravely. "They've tried to drown out the messages that tell me there's a lot wrong in my leg, but they don't seem to know how to hunt for the cause."

The cause of his sciatica was unusual. It took two days of constantly living with the man to discover why his case was so stubborn and uncommonly severe. But when once found, the treatment was the quintessence of good sense—and one that anyone can do at home as well as I did for Dr. Roberts in Mexico.

HOW TO STRETCH THE LEG TO RELIEVE NERVE PRESSURE

While hunting for the reason for Dr. Roberts' unusual leg pains, it seemed wise to rid his system of all the irritants and toxins he'd accumulated over the years. With papayas plentiful in Mexico, I had the sufferer eating scarcely anything more than this fruit for three days. Because the papaya contains a valuable protein enzyme, this diet dug deeply into the man's tissues and digested down to normal end-products the accumulated protein toxins that were nipping at his nerve-endings. This alone was able to still the leg pains better than the salicylates he had been taking—and without side effects.

Meanwhile, Dr. Roberts could find no position at all that gave him relief. Then the idea came to me. Could it be that the sciatic nerve itself was rubbing against the bony rim of the notch that it had to pass through? It turned out that this was the case. And exactly this happens in many cases of sciatica that are not easily helped by customary techniques. In that event, stretching the involved leg does the required job.

To find a position—any position—that offered relief, I requested the suffering man to lie down on the floor and rest his stockinged foot up against the wall. This was to reverse the down-pull of gravity. While he was lying thus, close to the wall with leg straight up on the wall, I told him to lock his knee and reach upward on the wall as high as possible. This he did with surprising ease. Now I instructed him to kind of inch in with his seat closer and closer to the wall, meanwhile reaching his leg higher on the wall, stretching it to the full. We both learned that the farther up he reached the more it stilled the pain in his leg.

Finally, Dr. Roberts worked his good leg into a curled-under position and was able to have his involved leg stretched rigidly straight up against the wall. He held this a moment or two, then a deep sigh of relief issued from him. "Doctor," he cried with the thrill of discovery. "Doctor, this does it! I've got no pain at all—for the first time!"

By stretching the muscles of the involved leg, the big, fat, very long sciatic nerve had also been inched toward the center of the sciatic notch. No longer did the most tender of all human tissue, nerve tissue, rub against the hardest of all tissue, the bony rim of the sciatic notch. Once away from contact and friction, the nerve pain subsided. And once knowing this technique, the suffering Dr. Roberts was in control of his future worries. He knew what to do. Being cautioned that this was not by any means a cure but only a relief measure—that we had only found the mechanically right way to lift pressure off his sciatic nerve—he was handed the complete Missing Link program and went on his way. Later he reported that the improved and newly developed Missing Link techniques proved a revelation to him in improved general health.

HOW ANOTHER PERSON CAN HELP
YOU STRETCH YOUR LEG

Living against gravity as we do, lying on the floor and resting your legs against the wall occasionally is an approved form of gravity-reversal. Also, getting someone to stretch your leg from time to time can be rewarding, restful, and helpful in preventing future trouble.

Here's how it's done. As you lie on your back at the edge of a bed, your spouse or friend can raise your leg and place your heel on his shoulder. If the shoulder is too high, he bends down for this. While thus crouching to accommodate your Achilles tendon on his shoulder, your helper curls the toes of your foot *inward,* toward your shinbone. He does this with one hand; and the leg-stretch is felt at once. Now, with the other hand, he forces the bent knee into a locked position. This straightens the leg and stretches it further. For a final and full stretch, the helper raises himself out of the crouch into standing position, taking your leg upward with him. The forced stretch may give temporary discomfort. Try to stand it for a moment or two. Then your helper will bend the knee of your leg and ease the pull at once. You stand up and feel taller, more limber, with more leg power as the immediate result of this technique.

HOW TO RESHAPE SHAPELESS LEGS

Little Gloria, age 9, was a blonde, blue-eyed child with the face of an angel. But she had heavy, shapeless legs that looked like cylinder posts; legs that neither curved out at the calves nor tapered down at the ankles. And she was a lifelong epileptic, having had at least one seizure of epilepsy per week since the beginning of her pathetic life.

Were I an internist with the specialty of hunting down fancy and bedazzling labels for human ailments, I could have spent half a lifetime determining precise diagnoses for Gloria's problems. But happily I was trained to go at human maladies *naturally* and not waste time in seeking names, diagnoses, labels. Was little Gloria's central problem essentially glandular? Was it of nervous origin? Did it taper down to a digestive hook-up? Or was it due to not just one, but many different causes? These frighteningly time-wasting matters would have occupied the conventional diagnostician. But my way was different; a different *examination,* a different *approach,* a different *method,* hopefully a different outcome—vastly different *results.*

Examination. I found pressures on nerves at the base of the neck, also at the very last vertebrae of the spine, and also in the feet themselves. These I adjusted into normal position, then showed them how to do all this for themselves; and gave instructions informing Gloria and her mother how to keep the body from accumulating any new nerve-pinching problems. The child loved the Head-Lift and Pelvic Back-Tip and Squat Drills which achieved these results.

Approach. With the nerves being free to deliver to the legs the Life Force needed for function and self-repair, my approach was now to reshape the legs themselves, and also see to it that there was adequate nerve supply in the feet as such.

Method. To reshape the feet and at the same time assure a non-pinched flow of nerve impulses, my method was the ROLLING PIN drills each night at bedtime. To give new shape to the legs, however, the method was a two-fold one. Toe-raising in a pigeon-toed position. Gloria stood with feet about six inches apart and "toed in," which means bringing the toes so close together that they almost touched. From this position my instruction was to raise herself rapidly and vigorously on her toes—up and down, up and down until very tired in the calves. This kept raising the bones of the arches and also tightening the muscles of the legs. Rocking back and forth on her feet—from way back on both heels to far forward on all toes—until quite tired. All this followed by a warm (not hot) footbath and a 15-minute rest with feet elevated on pillows.

Results. Once those post-like legs of hers began taking form and shape, there was no holding the child back. She wanted to do too much, in fact. But it was a plus-thing, a new mental outlook that lifted her to high elevation, quite a change from the former self-hatred due to the epilepsy.

No After-Dinner Leisurely Strolls

I learned that she had what the family thought was the "healthy habit" of taking a leisurely after-dinner stroll. The idea, they said, was to "work the food down." I stopped this, explaining that to digest the meal the stomach needs the blood right there in its own area, not dispersed to the muscles used in walking. Watch the animals *in nature.* After a meal they curl up and rest. This had the result of improving Gloria's digestion and elimination. Moreover, when the mother told me that the child had a "nice cozy electric blanket every night," I stopped this also. "Her body was made to generate the heat she needs," I explained. "If you produce artificially what the body ought to manufacture naturally, then in time she will become debilitated. *What you don't use, you lose.* Nature takes away those functions that you don't employ." All this was new to them; but so is the usual natural approach, and method of healing, to people weaned and reared on artificial, unnatural doctoring ways.

Avoid the Use of Electric Blankets

A further word about electric blankets. I do not mean to indicate they are entirely bad. Do not throw them away on my say-so. But I do mean that they should not be used *all* night. Using an electric blanket for a few minutes before retiring can be a fine way of making the sheets toast-warm, so one doesn't have to experience the shock of crawling in between icy sheets. But once in bed, my advice is to turn off the current and use the blanket merely as a cover, not as a heating device. Let your own body do the job it was intended to do. If you stoke the bodily furnace artificially, it will forget how to do it naturally.

As to Gloria, her epileptic seizures lessened in severity and in frequency. Under the complete *Missing Link* program of countering gravity strains, reoxygenating the body and detoxifying the blood-stream (see *Glossary*), she finally withdrew entirely from dependence on bromides and phenobarbital. Even the few pimples from the bromides evaporated and she was pleased pink with her looks. The final hurdle to jump was the extraction of a few bad molars. I telephoned the dentist to give her gas rather than an injection, and then to refer her back to me immediately, for I feared that if anything would kick off another epileptic "fit" after freedom from them for three months, the dental work might. She came back in fine fettle. I watched her for another week and discharged her. I hadn't known what an effusive child she really was, for up to then Gloria acted quietly dignified—or had the "shame pattern" of some epileptics. But when I told her she was discharged, needing no more visits or treatments, she threw her little arms around me and kissed me emotionally. The taste of that kiss still lingers.

HOW TO TREAT A PAINFUL TAILBONE

Now I ought to tell you how to treat a painful tailbone—that remaining remnant of a "monkey's tail" that hangs onto the end of our spine.

Captain Gordon was a professional ship's pilot who guided seagoing vessels out of the harbor into open waters. Several years before I saw him, during a shipping strike of some kind, he was mistaken on a dark pier for a strikebreaker and beaten by rough men within an inch of his life. During the beating, his coccyx (tailbone) was kicked by heavy boots and broken into several pieces. When I saw him, Captain Gordon hadn't been able to sit down "square on the back of his lap" for more than two years. The way he sat was with one buttock on a chair and the remainder of him hanging over empty space. He was in constant, excruciating pain. His wife had to accompany him on each visit.

He was a heavy man. Also quite rich. And a man who'd seen the "best doctors" and spent a tidy fortune seeking help.

I hardly knew where to start. An X-ray of his tailbone showed it to be a shattered-to-bits affair rather than a bone in one piece. So I played it safe by advising the absolutely natural things that always helped, no matter what the problem.

Knowing that he ate the fancy "unfoods" that they served him out of "The Captain's Mess" when he piloted a ship—sometimes for as long as two days at a stretch without a wink of sleep—I began by insisting that he follow the *List of Foods and Drinks to Avoid* (see page 84). Then, the first time he was free of piloting duties, he had a detoxifying physiological rest by way of a three-day fast. This was followed by a full week of monodiet because he also needed to lose weight.

Meanwhile the nerve pressures in his lower spine that I'd discovered were correctively treated and he was given corrective home drills to follow. (See *Glossary.*) All those on hands and knees he could do with ease and surprisingly great benefit. These were the Sway and Arch, Knee-Chest and Head Hang over the bed's edge. So while new and uninterrupted nerve impulses were flowing to the tailbone by means of the self-repairing Life Force characteristic of nerve impulses (all resulting from correcting his nerve pressures in the low spine), the counter-gravity drills were making up for other physical indignities to his body over the years. The newly upgraded and purified blood stream was detoxified through his diet, thus the former toxic accumulations no longer "bit" into and irritated his nerve-endings. He was prepared for the specific work.

His wife was taught the technique of applying hot-cold-hot sprays to his lower buttock and coccygeal area. And, very carefully, I entered his rectum with a well-lubricated rubber glove to begin dilating the anal spincters and straightening out his shattered tailbone from the inside.

HOW TO USE THE HOT-COLD-HOT
TECHNIQUE TO ELIMINATE PAIN

The great thing in the captain's case was pain. It was constant and unrelenting. How could he get that pain quieted so he could live with it?—that was his everlasting question. So I had a talk with "Lady Gordon." She was the man-behind-the-gun in the case. "Do you know what a bathspray is?" I asked her. Sure, they used one on her hair in the beauty parlor for shampooing, it was a spray-head at the end of a long rubber hose. "Well, have the captain stand up in the bathtub and you spray water on his lower spine and bottom in hot-cold, hot-cold alternations." The technique took about 19 minutes to use. First, she sprayed hot water on the tailbone area for four minutes. It was to be as hot as he could comfortably stand. Then, without any in-between temperature, a spray of very cold water was to be aimed at his tissues for one minute. Another four minutes of hot, one of cold; then another four of hot and one of cold; finally, a spray of hot water for four minutes to finish the technique.

I believe in having any treatments I give accord *naturally* with the physiology of the body, and this hot-cold-hot technique does. (I vigorously oppose "shots" because they do not accord with natural physiological needs and perpetuate human disease, I am convinced, by polluting bloodstreams with foreign, diseased proteins which weaken resistance against future disease.) In this case the spray of very hot water brought about a blood vessel dilatation and rapid inflow of fresh blood nutrition to the surrounding tissues. Then, the sudden cold spray contracted the blood vessels and squeezed out the blood, together with its waste products. Then followed another surge of hot water and another dilatation accompanied by inrushing blood, with another contraction to send the blood away. In this way, we achieve a kind of pumping action: blood pumped in and out of the ailing part. The technique requires that we *begin with hot and finish with hot.* Thus the ailing parts are dilated at the end, and full of new rich blood.

An important note belongs here, I think. This exact technique sometimes helps cases of impotence when used *on the front* of the body. It cannot do harm, so should be tried. The trouble, I have learned, is that patients tend to consider this some kind of magic cure when it is really only a *meanwhile* thing—only something to help along until the program takes hold, for health is the result of a program (like the Missing Link program here given) rather than any magic button pushed anywhere on the body.

Following the hot-cold-hot spray technique, the captain's pain was so much diminished that he was able to lie flat on his back and do the important Abduct Thighs drill. After a few of these, he was instructed to do the Pelvic Back-Tip. These two drills opened the intervertebral spaces in his lower back, permitting a better and freer downflow of self-repairing energy to the hurting tailbone. With apprehension he tried the Primordial Walk and found he could do it. Then he was off and running toward health.

USE ONLY THE NEUTRAL BATH IN GREAT PAIN

The only bathing I permitted the captain to do was to submerge his body up to his neck in the Neutral Bath. (See *Glossary,* chapter 12, for this and all other techniques mentioned here.) I showed the "man-behind-the-gun" in the case, his solicitous and intelligent wife, how to hang a thermometer over the edge of the bathtub so it sits in the water suspended by a looped wire. "Get a water thermometer or even a plain ordinary one," I said. "The numbers will be magnified by the water; you'll read them easily when they hit around 99 degrees. Then his body will be suspended between equivalent temperatures—the same outside and inside his body—and everything that can relax will relax." I also instructed her how to insert a rectal dilator into the rectum while he was in the knee-chest position, resting thus for 15 minutes at a time. "I'll give you a professional dilator, but your own vaginal douche piece can also serve. Just lubricate it well and insert it with confidence; nothing to get hurt there."

With this home program the captain's pains continued to lessen, then were fairly wafted away completely. I recall the last afternoon of their visit, for Gordon's lady was always with him. "You two are ordered to go to a movie," I told them. "There's one in the shopping zone that has a matinee. You, Captain, are instructed to sit right back full on your natural seat for the full two hours, then report back to me for a re-check." He had not been able to sit on more than one buttock for years, but he did sit through this movie, and enjoyed it, with his weight flat down on buttocks and coccyx. The tailbone had welded its shattered pieces with natural cementum made inside the body by the body's own magical self-repairing factory. Now the captain understood me when I said my final word. *The power which created you is the power that can heal you.*

The big, highly-placed and very successful man stood there with tears in his eyes. He trembled as we shook hands. "In truth," he said, "I've achieved rejuvenated health." His body had, in fact, gone through a miracle tune-up.

HOW TO RELIEVE PAINFUL KNEES

Mrs. Julia Lowrie had the most curious knee problems I had ever seen. To obtain relief from the pain in her right knee she had to stand on one leg, the left one, like a pelican, with the right knee bent and the right ankle resting on the left thigh. "Thank God for banisters," she said. "I get so much pain walking down the staircase that if it weren't for the banisters I'd fall for certain."

That was the tip-off; pain when going *down* (not up) stairs. The shinbone had somehow been worked out of its normal position and the head of it had gone backward. The elderly lady was quite wealthy and had consulted "big men" who'd talked about semi-lunar cartilages and patellar ligaments and complex surgeries. All she needed was to have the tibial bone brought forward with a short, easy snap near the knee, then she walked with ease. The technique was easy. The human body tends toward the normal. That out-of-place tibial head just *wanted* to get back where it belonged. When I merely grasped it where it needed grasping and gave a little frontward jerk, it went into position at once. Now, it only needed explaining to the lady how to keep that knee from getting back into trouble.

First, she relaxed everything in a Neutral Bath. Then, lying on her back, she placed a pillow or a thick roll of towel under the right knee and carefully worked the shin backward toward the thigh. This used the roll or towel behind her knee as a kind of fulcrum which spread her knee-joint as she stretched the shinbone toward the thigh. *It did for her just about what I had done with my adjustment of her tibia.*

There was an amusing sequel to this. When I presented her with my bill she gasped. "Isn't that a steep fee for only a little thing you did on my knee and 20 minutes of advice?" she demanded. "No, it's for a lifetime of special study and experience," I told her. "What are you complaining of? Your trouble has been pinpointed and corrected. You have no pain there now. How much did you pay the others *without* relief, please tell me."

"H'mmm. Sounds right," she admitted. Then she wanted to know how this happened to her knee. "I don't know," I said. "You are a machine with many working parts in it, and you're active all the time. There are hundreds of ways a thing like this can be caused. All I know is what's there and what to do for it." Then I handed her the real shocker. "You are not cured, Mrs. Lowrie. I've shown you the mechanical aid to your knee problem. But the fact that your shinbone gave way at the knee shows a predisposing weakness. You need to follow a program—a tune-up miracle that your own body can perform for you. Do you care about rejuvenating your health?"

This was new to her, but she wanted all she could get that she'd paid for. I've disguised her name to save embarrassment, but if she reads this she will know herself in this story. From an over-rich and self-indulgent woman she became a star patient and a very healthy one.

Elements of the Missing Link Program

In her social circle she even became a kind of nuisance, the way she worked on people to observe the elements of the *Missing Link* program. Do the drills that make up for living against gravity, she urged. Get those pressures off nerves, for they interfere with the flow of Life Force to the sick parts of your body. Upgrade the ability of your system to oxygenate. Fast a little and then eat so that the body will eliminate the toxins in the blood. Relax properly with rectal dilatations and baths of body temperatures. The lady had it all.

HOW YOU CAN HELP HEAL
YOUR VARICOSE VEINS AT HOME

Henrietta Small was a young housewife with bulging varicose veins. She reported that even in adolescence she had signs of them, but after the birth of her two babies they began bulging and hurting. Surgical procedures were recommended, but she had a mortal dread of hospitals, of having the veins injected, dried out, stripped, and so forth. Besides the varicose condition, the woman had a recurring sacroiliac problem. Just bending over nearly killed her. She could hardly straighten out.

First things. first. I told her to go to a pool near her home *every day* and pick out the pool area no higher than her waistline. There, with water no higher than her middle, and thus no fear of drowning, she was to *run backwards*. Raise her knees high with each movement and race backwards with great vigor. Doing it, she felt the water slide over the calves of her legs like a hydro-therapy massage. She was counseled to continue running backward until quite tired, then rest in the Knee-Chest position. Following a 15-minute rest counter-gravitationally, another workout for her leg veins was advised.

"Lie flat on your back," I told her. "Place both feet on pillows for elevation and curl the toes inward toward the shinbones." This stretches the Achilles' tendons and works to reshape the legs, meanwhile acting to boost the tissues contiguous to the protruding veins. In just one week of attending diligently to this daily "home-work" Henrietta felt considerable relief.

But there was still a program to get started; for the local treatment did little to correct the systemic cause of her ill health. She still had her sacroliliac distress, scarcely able to straighten up after bending; she still had toxins (body poisons) in her system; she had nerve pressures to be released; she needed a good new reoxygenating program, as is common with every varicose case I have ever seen, and most certainly she needed to do a lot to overcome the effects of living against gravity. In her, merely from what I thought was a genetic weakness, counter-gravitational living had taken a greater toll than was usual in people her age.

Following my plan of first things first, the second item was to help the poor young woman straighten up like a human being after bending forward, as she had to very often with two babies. This was ridiculously easy.

HOW TO HELP YOURSELF OUT OF LOW BACK PAIN

"Reach around to the fold right under your buttocks," I advised. "That's called the gluteal fold, because those thick gluteal muscles fold inward to form the thighs at that point. Now, with your fingers reaching in back of you and hooked under those gluteal folds, just *lift them lightly*. Go ahead and try it." She bent forward, halted with pain on trying to stand erect, placed her fingers under the gluteal folds and lifted *gently*—very lightly—as I directed. Her spine straightened without pain and she smiled. "If this occurs at home, have your husband do it for you. By yourself, you now have the first-aid self-help answer."

On examination it was found that instead of the sacroiliac trouble she was supposed to have, it was not anything wrong between that flatiron-shaped sacral bone and her hip bones. It was a case of the last vertebra of her spine being jammed tight into the sacrum—what's called a lumbo-sacral lesion. Merely a few Pelvis Back-Tip drills that I taught her how to do (see *Glossary*) opened up the jammed area and gave her relief. Thus far we were dealing only with relief—a very dramatic lot of stuff that looked like fancy doctoring but wasn't at all anything like a cure. To get well, this young woman needed the entire *Missing Link* program, not merely sparkling little, magic-like, relief-changes. Lord knows, she needed her health to care for those infants she had.

Talk about pinched nerves! In Mrs. Small's neck, there was interference with the transmission of nerve power to all the rest of her body below. In tests for mobility, in turning the neck, she could turn the head all the way in one direction and just a fourth that distance in the other. Plenty of Head-Lift drills took care of that,

especially after I'd started correcting the nerve-root neck compressions with my own adjusting techniques in the office. Then she
was found to have whopping nerve pressures in her lower spine that
could easily have prevented the normal flow of power to her
varicosed legs. She was advised to *Hang from Loops* to stretch the
spine and separate the intervertebral discs. The Sway and Arch and
the Diaphragmatic Breathing drills helped her enormously. The
Dowager's Hump and especially the Primordial Walk returned her to
a state of general health, and she really felt *a miracle tune-up* taking
place in her body. Merely the addition of some attention to her diet
was what she needed. It did not appear wise to have her fast, since
she had the babies to attend to, but a long monodiet program
cleansed her bloodstream adequately.

THE FALLACY OF USING COMMERCIAL
ANTI-PERSPIRANTS

Quite by chance, I learned that Henrietta used anti-perspirants.
She sweated profusely, she said, and just had to do something. But I
pointed out the highly dangerous possibility of this practice and
advised her to stop it at once.

The skin is a breathing organ. It is an air-conditioning organ also.
It maintains the internal furnace at about 98.6 degrees Fahrenheit.
To shut out an endangering cold draft it closes tight to protect you,
and you can see the goose pimples. To let some excess heat out of
you on a hot day, it opens its million pores and sweats out the
excess. But it cannot do this if you commit a "crime" against it.
Deodorants are bad enough. But they are not anti-(against) perspiring
agents. They don't shut off the valves, close the sweating doors tight.
To put something that's dazzlingly advertised on your skin to fight
perspiration—to stop and block it—is a fallacy and serious health-
destroying act against yourself. When I see this and other com-
mercially induced "crimes" against life and health widely touted in
our nation, I wish I were the powerful head of HEW or FDA, one
with a free hand to serve the people instead of commercial interests.

Henrietta Small did all the things that were advised, and she did
them well. Her family was not noted for long-lived individuals, so she
did not expect to exceed what she called her "genetic inheritance."
Nevertheless, her formerly varicose-veined legs grew shapely, she had
no more pain in her spine at all, and—through unremitting Diaphragmatic Breathing, she said—her chest came up and her carriage
exhibited a woman of sparkling health.

A DRAMATIC BUT SIMPLE WAY
TO HELP ITCHING SKIN

The doctors call it pruritus. It can be nasty and drive one nearly wild. *Pruritus ani* means itching at the opening to the rectum, and victims have been known to scratch themselves into blood poisoning. Then there is pruritus of the vagina that's so fierce that at times women scratch the vulva, or outer lips, so hard that there's bleeding with no cessation of the itch at all.

HOW LOOKING GOOD CAN HIDE POOR HEALTH

Trudy was a fashion-plate young lady who looked very good but had health that was very poor indeed. She came into the office for cosmetic reasons. A purplish rash on her left leg just above her ankle could not be handled satisfactorily by the conventional doctors who prescribed drugs, and to this modern, style-conscious young lady it was the worst kind of torture to be thus marked. "Why can't I get something that hurts and is *hidden,* instead of this beastly something that doesn't hurt but gives me the mark of the beast?" she wailed. How little she knew the real sufferings of those with diseased inner viscera! However, she had her share of problems besides the leg rash.

The unbeautiful discoloration at her left ankle was what brought her in, but a rectal itch that just wouldn't quit was what drove her nearly frantic. The drug-prescribing allopaths she had consulted never even examined her lower spine, where the nerves come out of the spinal cord to feed Life Force to the anal and rectal area; thus they missed the cause altogether. She kept using one salve after another, those prescribed and those she merely heard about, and kept on scratching and suffering as best she could. When I corrected the nerve pressures which she was carrying around without knowing that she was, her itch diminished considerably but did not quit. Then I asked her what perfumes she used and instructed her to change the brand (for I'd learned years ago that sometimes the mere swapping of one poison for another helped these itching conditions). No help at all in that quarter. When Miss Elegant Trudy mentioned casually one day that she couldn't wait to get out of my office because "she was dying for a smoke," I got another idea.

"Look, Lady Elegance," I said to her. "I really shouldn't be putting up with the likes of you because you won't quit smoking those vile cigaroots, but . . . "

"But everybody puts up with the likes of me," she mimicked ingratiatingly, "because I *am* elegant and such an adornment."

"Well then," I temporized, "change your brand. That's one thing. In addition, change the habit-pattern of reaching for each cigarette."

I'm sure she thought me aberrated, but she indulged me. "You know how I corrected those nerve pressures in your back and the itch almost went away," I reminded her. "With the Sway and Arch and the Pelvic Back-Tip that I taught you to do, you could have corrected those nerve pressures yourself, or at least helped them a lot."

"Yes, and I still do them, so I'm a very good girl," she said, smiling her spoiled-brat, misbehaving smile.

"Now," I continued, "where do you keep your cigarettes at the office?" They were customarily in the top righthand drawer, she informed me. "Very well, then. First, you must change from this brand you smoke to another kind—any other you like. Second, keep the cigarettes in the lowermost *lefthand* drawer. Your habit-pattern is to reach into that top right drawer almost automatically. Let's un-gear you. Listen, now. When you feel you must absolutely take a cigarette, interrupt yourself for it. Get up from your chair, walk around your desk, sit down and take the pack from the side opposite to that you're accustomed to. If a smoke is worth that much, it's worth this extra effort. This will change the entire pattern of your smoking habit."

My motive behind these instructions was twofold. Just by changing her brand she might get rid of that worrisome *pruritus ani*—and she did. It was dramatic. After the first day of taking a new kind of poison aboard, what was left of the itch went away. She was astonished, and certainly most gratified. But the other part of it also worked. I knew that she smoked a lot more than she would if the cigarettes were hard to reach. It was too easy—and far too automatic—to reach into the accustomed drawer and *take a cigarette out of sheer habit,* not even when she desired one, often not even aware that she was reaching for one. So by reconditioning her pattern, especially when I forbade her carrying cigarettes in her purse on the street but only, if necessary, a couple stashed away in her bosom, she reported smoking half her usual amount. Less poison entering her system, less toxins to disturb her. Later, with a lot of Diaphragmatic Breathing drills, her system was aerated and reoxygenated to the point where she lost her desire for smoking altogether.

HOW TO GET RID OF AN ATTACK OF HICCUPS

Our super-elegant Lady Trudy was free of her *pruritus ani* but, as mentioned, still in very bad health despite very good looks. Her discolored leg had not abated. She had frontal sinusitis, with pains in her forehead above her eyes so agonizing at times that she felt her head would blow off. From time to time, she thought she would die from attacks of hiccups that continued around the clock and weakened her, causing a quick and severe loss of weight. The list was imposing. To make herself see herself clearly, I ordered her to write her problems down, hoping in this way to win her full cooperation in observing the *Missing Link* program. One day she handed me the list. *The True Trudy List,* was how she headed it.

1. Itch: you-know-where. Now gone, praise be!

2. Rash above left ankle. Nasty purple, not Royal Purple. I'm in a purple passion to get rid of it, please sir.

3. Hiccups every whipstitch. Makes my tummy plop up and my weight plop away. Can't I manage to stay at my oh-so-nice 110?

4. Sinus attacks: when it hits me I get crosseyed. Unprettily so.

5. Can't hold urine. Sometimes I "tinkle" when excited, as in sex.

About the frequent hiccup attacks our young lady was really scared, in spite of her endeavor at sophisticated indifference. She had one while at the office, which was ideal. Taking an ice-cube out of the small office refrigerator, I placed it on top of her collarbones, first one and then the other. The ice slid behind the clavicle (collarbone) into the groove between the bone and the neck. That's where the main nerve supply passes on its way to the diaphragm, and the diaphragm is the offending organ in hiccups. The quick contact of ice causes the nerve to contract; the nerve impulses cannot flow through to the diaphragm temporarily because we've frozen the nerve pathway for a minute; without nerve impulses the diaphragm quits doing its plop-plop hiccuping. Bingo—no more attacks.

I say that Trudy's attack at the office was ideal. Perhaps I should say fortuitous. In this way she learned what to do to stop the hiccups. Knowing this, she was mentally relieved, no longer frightened, for she knew that a prolonged hiccups seizure can wear a person down to his death. Now the ice-freezing technique gave her comfort. Oddly, however, she never again had a hiccups attack and any use for her new-found knowledge.

WHEN THE SHOTS HAVE BEEN MANY
THE FASTING MUST BE LONG

The reader is already aware of my deep aversion to injections, speaking purely as a doctor. Trudy had taken many drugs and shots. I told her that I believed human disease is perpetuated by drugs and especially shots which *pollute human bloodstreams and weaken resistance against disease*. Outside of a rare shot of morhpine, for instance, in the most extreme of emergencies (as when a leg has been almost severed in an accident and one would die of the unbearable pain), I am not in favor of shooting foreign protein products, nearly always diseased products, into human bodies in the name of healing those bodies.

With the loss of her pruritus and attacks of hiccups, Trudy was getting well. But there was yet much left to do. Not least of what remained to do was purifying the young woman's bloodstream, getting the accumulated, uneliminated toxins out of her body. I had no great worry about the rash on her left leg; long ago I'd discovered that dermatology problems were digestive at base, and if I could upgrade her elimination through the regular eliminative channels the skin would not need to lend a hand. So I made the elegant young sophisticate face up to the real needs of the case, otherwise I declared that this time I would wash my hands of her. "I want to succeed on this case, not fail on it," I warned her sternly. "Therefore don't you dare make me fail by ignoring my instructions, severe as they may seem to you." Having already seen more results than she expected, she promised to go along.

BENEFITS OF THE FAST

To begin with, she needed an absolute fast—and for the kind of young lady she was, this was anathema. "I'll lose weight," she began, then halted in her complaints when she saw I would abide no more pouting immaturity. Because she had had a great many shots for a great variety of troubles, her bloodstream was laden with foreign toxins. This necessitated a long fast—a real, uninterrupted physiological rest. I explained what this entailed.

"But what do I do all that time?" she asked with a plea in her voice.

"Nothing," I said. "Just absolutely nothing."

HOW TO DO NOTHING INTELLIGENTLY

For all her spoiled ways this young woman was not lacking in intelligence. When I outlined to her the deep meaning and healing philosophy behind "doing nothing intelligently," she got the idea. Years ago in college I'd had a professor who hammered this at his students. "Get the idea, then all else follows," he would say. (Trudy absorbed the idea of doing nothing intelligently, realizing that the bodily energies employed in daily functions could be conserved by a period of no eating, no talking, reading, walking, writing letters, listening to radios, and so forth. All this energy usually employed in digesting foods, and in taking us through our daily routines could now be centered on repairing the damages the body had accumulated.) "Why, the heart alone beats more than a hundred thousand times a day, and the volume of blood it pumps in two weeks (the period I wanted her to fast and do nothing except lie in bed) is more than twenty-five thousand gallons. If you listen to the wisdom of the body—as an animal does when it just lies down and does nothing, during illness—you have no idea now what good health you may enjoy later throughout all your future. Wouldn't you love to have a leg clear of splotchy rashes?"

That last tipped the scale. Trudy went to bed and stayed there for two weeks, sipping only distilled water when thirsty. She was permitted only a 15-minute period in the sun daily for a nude sunbath—giving her a vitamin D meal thereby—and lying on her back on the floor with her legs resting high up against the wall. "If you're going to tear a two-week period out of your life for your long future health, let's do it exactly right," I counseled, "no matter what the sacrifice. A bit of sacrifice now in exchange for good health hereafter sounds all right to me, doesn't it to you?"

She agreed, and followed instructions faithfully despite the loss of ten pounds during the two weeks. After the fast she had nothing but lightly steamed zucchini squash for one day, in order to accustom her to foods. Zucchini, unseasoned as it was, tasted better to the young woman than any food she had ever had before in her life. At times, I have advised breaking a fast with a day or two of fruit-juice. But on occasion, people react unfavorably to the juice's acidity. Never, however, have I found anyone to react unfavorably to mild, tender zucchini. It is merely steamed for a few minutes and then insalivated thoroughly—meaning chewed until it is all fluid.

I had learned in the course of this that Trudy used anti-perspirants regularly. "What! And stop the skin from breathing out its wastes! Stop it from sweating out its toxins!" Quite meekly she asked what she could use instead.

HOW TO MAKE YOUR OWN NATURAL DEODORANT

While she was on a long monodiet program following the fast, Trudy was sent to a health food store and bought a bottle of tiny chlorophyll tablets. These were nothing more than compressed alfalfa, flaxseed, and other greens. When one tablet went into a jar of water it turned the fluid green. This can be used for mouth-gargling, if desired; and if an underarm deodorant is needed several tablets dissolved in water make up a fine natural deodorizing product.

Trudy's neck was a mass of nerve pressures. These I corrected, but she could have done the same for herself (or very nearly as well) by means of the Head-Lift and Dowager's Hump and Sway and Arch programs (see *Glossary*). In all cases, the drills given here for releasing nerve pressures are very helpful, even when not as completely corrective as the treatments of a trained doctor of chiropractic, for example. With only the rarest of exceptions they improve the existing condition. Nearly always, they fully work the impingements away and leave the nerve pathway free to transmit its life force to the sick and deprived organs without interference. Therefore, the reader is advised most sincerely, consult the *Glossary* frequently and do the drills diligently, for it is the road to freedom from pinched nerves and the many diseases caused thereby.

HOW TO LOOK INTO YOUR OWN SINUS AREAS

When the angry purplish blotch in her leg finally faded away, Trudy also reported the end of her sinus problem. Formerly, I had shown her how to "throw light on the subject." In the office, I had cold white lights to transilluminate various areas: sinuses, breasts, teeth (to see if abscesses were forming long before the X-ray could pick them up), mastoids and even intra-uterine tumors or cysts. In Trudy's case, however, I made it simple by using an ordinary little flashlight, the slim pencil-type used for throat illumination and also sold in the dime stores. Darkening the room, I sat her in front of a mirror and pushed the end of the flashlight up alongside her nose under the corner of her eyebrows. The frontal sinus space showed up with black and dark-brownish splotches when she still had her sinus trouble; then, with the elimination of nerve pressures and with detoxifying her body, we did it again. Her sinuses were beautiful! A nice shade of pink, even all over, with nary a darkish spot anywhere.

This can be done at home to see your own maxillary sinuses also. In a dark room, the flashlight is placed inside the mouth upon the upper gums just under the cheekbone. The color will be a beautiful pink when healthy. If the sinuses are congested, you can expect to see dark colorations throughout the lighted area.

As you attend to getting better nerve supply into the area of the sinuses through doing the Head-Lift and Primordial Walk, plus getting better general oxygenation by way of Diaphragmatic Breathing and pushing up on the cheekbones where they join the nose (as given in chapter 1), you will find the sinus areas becoming a more beautiful pink. This indicates they are getting clear of foreign debris. A further great help will come from eliminating the mucus-forming foods also, as set forth in this volume.

In much the same way, a woman can see her breasts in a dark room with a strong light placed under the breasts, one at a time. The white cold light should be directed upward from under the breast, and as you look down you can see the network of blood vessels plus any lumps that may be forming.

HOW TO CONTROL A LEAKING BLADDER

Lady Trudy, in her inimitably spoiled way, had written on her list that she needed to urinate often, adding that sometimes she "tinkled when excited," especially during the sex act. This happens in women more often than is thought. The female bladder, for one thing, is considerably larger than the male bladder, containing about 400 cc. against the male's 250 cc. Thus, when the bladder is very full and a weight is over it as in sex, the valve may open during the heights of orgasm and a few drops of urine may "tinkle" out.

Man makes the mistake of holding back his desire to urinate or evacuate stools. Society forces this upon us. In the natural state, all animals urinate and defecate immediately when the urge comes upon them. But we humans bring about a long-continued irritation to the mucous membrane lining of the bladder by holding ourselves in when "we want to go." Eventually, the valve may weaken from over-long acid contact at the site of the valve due to not evacuating the urine when needed. Therefore I advise "going" as often as possible. Not "saving it up" until you are absolutely forced to void the bladder. Also, it is advisable not to drink anything several hours before retiring.

HOW TO HANDLE YOUR INSOMNIA
ALL BY YOURSELF WITHOUT DRUGS

Doctors often use the word *hyperemia,* which means too much blood in any part of the body. Its opposite is *anemia,* which denotes too little blood in any part. (Anemia has other meanings too, but for our purposes this is good enough, and useful.)

Now, what is the meaning of sleep? Sounds like a silly question—surely not one that's been asked frequently. Well, sleep is in a way a temporary anemia of the brain and a hyperemia of the body. Until the parts inside your cranium are *relatively* poor in blood, you cannot drift off to sleep. So long as you are thinking or planning or excited with any kind of conversation, the brain is rich with blood and you can't sleep. The brain is hyperemic—it has too much blood for sleep. But when the blood from the brain enters the body below—making the body hyperemic while the brain becomes anemic—you are free to relax, let go your thinking functions and tensions, and fall asleep.

How then can we help our own insomnia, since we know this? Easy, really. If you place a cold cloth to your forehead, it tends to contract the vessels in the head, which drives the blood out. It is known that the blood-flow follows heat; therefore, if you place a hot water bottle at the feet the blood will follow the heat, drifting away from the brain toward the body. You see? Knowledge is power, as this small example shows.

Trudy's active mind made her an insomniac, so when she understood this she knew how to help herself. No more counting sheep, which, she now could understand, was merely a way of boring the brain and driving the active blood out of it. Since calcium is known to be an agent to relax and untense the body, drinking warm milk at bedtime often helps the insomnia victim. Another cheery item to use is honey. A teaspoonful of honey sipped slowly, a drop at a time licked off the spoon, sometimes brings on sleepfulness better than anything else we know.

AN EXPLOSIVE NEW IDEA ABOUT BLOOD TRANSFUSIONS

One day I was showing Miss Trudy how to do the Bicycle-Aloft drill, the one I recommend for cardiac patients to increase their pulse-rate gradually and safely. In her case, I had her on the floor of my consulting room circling her raised legs around in order to keep her legs trim and free of future rashes, when she mentioned casually that some years earlier she needed a great many blood tranfusions. Now I saw another reason for her deep toxicity. I had seen it so often among those who'd had many blood transfusions.

I seriously question the alleged need of blood transfusions. Like the widely touted "shots" that the vast majority of doctors use, I question very much the data that's been assembled in favor of giving a patient another person's blood. Are we slaves to data? Data assembled by people who may have a personal and profit-motivated interest in our accepting it? Is there no other, and possibly better, way of treating the patient deficient in blood?

Some years ago, I helped in a small way to assemble and organize book material for a famous doctor who had never written a book and wanted help in getting his first one under way. It was Dr. Alonzo Shadman, a foremost and illustrious homeopath who had a hospital in which he did the surgery for a few hundred non-operating physicians. We had some correspondence and I gave him a little help in assembling material for his book.

Now this outstanding man had performed over twenty thousand surgical operations in some fifty years of surgery. One day he stopped using blood transfusions entirely and gave transfusions of normal saline solution instead. He reasoned that life came originally from the sea; therefore injecting pure salt water in the proper blood-like concentration (normal saline solution) would start up the body's own blood-manufacturing processes. He wrote to me that since changing from blood transfusions to saline solutions he had never lost a patient from lack of blood, "even when they were brought in chalk-white and exsanguinated," meaning that they were white from great loss of blood.

Now what is it exactly that I have against blood transfusions—I, a doctor for more than 40 years who has been listening to "the wisdom of the body" and observing natural rather than artificial methods of healing?

STARTLING FACTS ABOUT THE BLOOD

I believe with all my heart and physiological knowledge that the Bible is right when it declares that "the life is in the blood." All your inherited traits are there. In the blood are the buried personality traits: tendencies toward rheumatism, heart disease, lung ailments, lasciviousness or even wild adventurousness; tendencies toward drunkenness and kleptomania and claustrophobia and agorophobia and whatever else you wish to name. When you take on another's blood, you are taking on another's weaknesses and traits and habit patterns. It is not overstating the case when I say that many drunkards on "Skid Row" sell their blood at $5 a pint to obtain new drinking money. In slum areas of New York I have seen signs in store windows asking passersby to donate blood: *payment spot cash.* You have no idea, when you receive a blood transfusion, whether the blood came from one of your own race or background or temperament; and even when it comes from one of your own family you may be getting loaded onto you the immeasurable and presently undetectable "ultramicroscopie" toxins and patterns inimical to your well-being.

EVEN BABIES BECOME FOREIGN OBJECTS
AT THE END OF NINE MONTHS

Unmistakably, the human body exhibits an inner rejection mechanism, as in rejecting transplanted hearts, that ought to be observed with respect. The body does not want foreign cells injected into the system. If forced, as with "shots" and transfusions, it will somehow rise to the occasion and *appear* to accept what is thrust upon it. But when it can, it rejects anything foreign dumped into the system. A splinter in your finger is foreign; and the body works it up, and out, if at all possible. A fragment in your eye is washed out by the tears. The fetus at 280 days becomes a foreign object, because it can then breathe and eat on its own, and the labor mechanism starts up—a rejection mechanism that thrusts the fetus out of the body.

Just as, apparently, no doctors disapprove shots, so none disapproves blood transfusions. But we needn't accept their data blindly. With saline transfusions, the blood-making apparatus of the body itself is started up—and no foreign blood is needed. If the widely accepted data were truly dependable, it seems, we would not be having our present increases—rather than diminutions—in heart disease, cancer, mental illness, cerebral palsy, diabetes, arthritis, kidney degenerations, multiple sclerosis, muscular dystrophy, epilepsy, cystic fibrosis, and so on.

ARE YOU A DATA SLAVE?

The elegant Lady Trudy wondered whether some of her personality traits had come from the blood transfusion she'd had. The "turkey skin," for instance, which is how she referred to the recently sagging skin of her neck, which had just begun to show. "Is that a personality trait, Dr. Morrison, or an old-age characteristic?" she wanted to know. I advised her to do an exercise that I knew she would *over*-do, being the beauty-oriented lady she was. It consisted of pronouncing aloud the syllables "Oooooh-Eckus," "Oooooh-Eckus" over and over again. These are the Spanish pronunciations of the letters "U" and "X." If she held her hand lightly against the underskin of her jaw and neck while pronouncing these letters, she could feel, beyond doubt, the tremendous workout the skin got in this way.

While performing her "Oooooh-Eckus" drills one day she asked about my frequent reference to "data slaves." This lady wanted to know everything. For all her concentration on beauty and fashion, Trudy had the makeup of a researcher, a questing quality I respected highly in her.

I answered that one large fault I'd found with people in their relation to health-seeking was that they accepted data thrust at them by purportedly "scientific sources" or "authoritative quarters." Why didn't people think things through *themselves?*, I argued. Many ordinary people have excellent analytical intelligence. Many brainy people in top educational or technological positions, nevertheless, left their brains elsewhere when they accepted wholly, without personal analysis, some of the healing balderdash and flapdoodle handed them as solemn truth.

Most of the data you're handed may not stand the light of analysis or inspection. They may be utterly false while *seeming* to be true. The data may be to somebody's interest that you accept.

Popular Data Delusions Impairing Health

The schoolteacher warns the playing child. *Don't run, Johnny, or you'll get hot and catch cold.* The child was exercising his muscles, racing his blood, oxygenating his system, on the way to catch health, not catch cold. Even those who believe in pathogenic germs as causative factors also believe that resistance is what keeps germs from making a successful invasion of the body, and Johnny was building healthy resistance by running.

Don't work too hard or you'll keel over and drop dead. That's what solicitous friends were telling Jim as they passed him working hard and singing at his work. He didn't even know he was working *hard.* He was enjoying what he was doing and singing while doing it. But enough people warned him, with *the usual data* about the harmfulness of working hard, so that he began to worry about it and quit singing, quit enjoying his work, and worried himself into sickness.

Drink eight glasses of water a day. Even otherwise qualified doctors have splashed such data onto unknowing lay people who expected them to know. But people are not car radiators. Loads of water ought not be thrust down to overwork human kidneys. Where did the water-filling data come from? Nobody knows for sure.

Be sure to eat the skins of potatoes and apples and all—that's the best part. There you have data repeated by everyone. But is the skin the best part? Do we have enzymes strong enough to "cook down" fully anything as tough as apple skins? Why not the part of the apple near the center where the seeds are? After all, those seeds are the life-giving part of the fruit. The skins are so tight-woven, as protectively impermeable coveralls for the fruit or vegetable inside, that they may not be intended to be eaten, but to be peeled away. Haven't all of us noticed tomato skins, *undigested,* in our stools?

If you're catching cold all the time, better take shots for it. Which pharmaceutical firms started such data going? On top of the toxins already resident in the blood you're advised to add the protein wastes, usually diseased, from outside. And millions of data slaves do what they're instructed to do by the "scientific community," meaning those who advise it. ("We who give drugs and shots are the scientific community exclusively; if you don't believe it, just ask us.")

Better run and have a diagnosis to find out what you've got. Data slaves, who are really concerned well-wishers at the same time, assume that the doctors *can* reach a dependable diagnosis, not knowing that the odds are against it. On top of this, they assume that "of course a doctor cannot do anything for you unless he knows what's the matter with you," which is another slick datum that sounds so beautifully, unassailably right but happens to be dangerously and misleadingly and very time-wastingly wrong. While "Doc" uses up time hunting a diagnosis with his method, another with natural methods seeks out the nerve supply to the ailing part, removes nerve interferences in order to assure a free flow of healing energy to the part, and employs other natural means of helping the body to heal itself—regardless of whether a diagnostic label has been made, made wrongly, or not made at all.

The doctors are doing everything that's possible, but they're not winning the battle. But are they doing "everything possible"? Whose data is that? *Everything* possible would mean also everything that doctors who've been trained in other methods (than drug-and-shot-giving methods) can do. Their examinations and approaches and treatments are different, with possibly different results. If the natural, non-drugging doctors are not being consulted or used, not "everything" is being done, is it? If only one single method of approach—the allopathic method—is employed, then it is manifestly untrue to say that *everything possible* is being done. Yet the nation is awash with data slaves who believe that in such circumstances (as when a patient is failing or otherwise not rallying), the pronouncement that *everything possible* is being done means in fact that everything is.

HOW TO REASON YOURSELF OUT OF BECOMING A DATA SLAVE

The fashionable Miss Trudy, after so many drug prescriptions, shots, and transfusions, was finished with the old ways. Finished forever, she said extravagantly, "with what didn't give me health, and on the side of what did." She was in dead earnest.

"No more tinkering with my body chemistry . . . I'll let the body itself do it," is how the remarkable young lady put it. She understood, at last, that the body knows how: how to balance its own individual chemistry if given the smallest chance by way of natural methods inherent in the Missing Link program.

MONUMENTAL STEPS TO TUNING UP YOUR HEALTH

First, Step One, making up for the counter-gravitational ills of living in the perpendicular state, against gravity. Second, Step Two, unblocking all nerve pressures which interfere with the free conductivity of energizing and healing impulses to the ailing parts. Third, Step Three, insuring the proper and wholly natural blood chemistry through the medium of *fasting,* and *feeding,* and *avoiding,* in the department of food consumption. Fourth, Step Four, giving the entire system a new burst of energy, and a new miracle tune-up of rejuvenation, by way of Diaphragmatic Breathing and the like. Last, even with all these factors working for you, when fatigue creeps in, as it will at times, eliminating tensions and nerve-depleting enervations by means of the Neutral Bath and other aids such as Anal Dilatation.

Toward the end of our time together as patient and doctor, Trudy told me how she had reasoned herself out of being a data slave for all time to come. Said this erstwhile sophisticate: "I'll never again believe what the self-acclaimed scientists tell me, so long as they knock other doctors as being unscientific. If they were truly scientific, our diseases would be vanishing and the worth of the doctors would be self-evident. After all, the great man does not expect the field all to himself—without any competition. So long as those doctors don't want competitive doctors in the hospitals and clinics—just as though the hospitals belonged to them instead of being supported with everybody's tax money—I'm going to suspect them. Suspect their motives as well as their claim to being so ultra-scientific."

I was listening to unassailable logic out of the mouth of one who had been flippantly un-serious just a short while back, when, as she put it, "I enjoyed all that miserable health in place of this present good health."

She placed her hands on her hips and the spark of the evangelist came into her eyes.

"There's been every imaginable kind of drug around," she said. "They're trying to sell a zillion drugs to us out of every TV set and paper and magazine every day. Every imaginable kind for balancing our blood chemistry, our body chemistry and what-all. Well, if just balancing our inside chemistry were *enough*, we'd have almost no cancer or heart disease, or all those mentally sick people crowding the hospitals, and all those contributions asked from us because so many diseases are rising all the time. The way you say it yourself," she said, addressing me, "If drugs cure, why does anyone die except of old age?" She took a deep breath and finished in high altitude. "Yessirree, brother. If drugs really cured people, with all the scads of 'em around and new ones kept coming at us, nobody except the very old ones would ever, ever die."

CHAPTER NINE

How to Compensate
for the Strain of Living Against Gravity
to Rejuvenate Your Health

Human beings have serious health problems that can be traced directly to something you've probably never heard about. That "something" that you never hear mentioned is gravity. Yes, gravity. It pounds down our organs and tissues every day. It's the great unspoken, unmentioned major cause of human disease. How to cope with this health destroyer is dealt with in this chapter.

We human beings live every second of every day with the constant unhealthy down-pull of gravity against us. Our limbs, our chest organs, our abdominal organs, all are weighted down and forced to work ceaselessly *uphill* to cope with the effects of gravity; not on a horizontal plane, like the animal's. The animal's body rests squarely and well-balanced upon "all fours." His four legs form posts that are stationed firmly, and more or less equally, upon the ground. But we human beings—well, every waking moment of our lives we must bear, consciously or unconsciously, the strains and stresses of living against gravity that is working against our health.

This enormously important factor has not been evaluated or even noticed in the doctoring professions. It's been *missing* from their thinking. How can doctors afford to miss anything so obviously contributive in the field of disease causation? That is the big, extraordinary question. But it is not *our* question: our field of interest is *the answer*, the answer to what has been the heretofore unnoticed but all-too-obvious cause of strains and stresses on the human organism. There you have the *Missing Link* in doctoring—until now.

To be well, absolutely every one has to compensate for the daily stressful down-pull of gravity on his organs. If he misses doing this he is doomed to be sick in some ways, and in some degree. There is just no way to escape it. To doctor anyone without prescribing compensations for gravitational strains on the body is only half-doctoring in my opinion, an opinion stemming from 40 years of research in the field.

So what I propose to do in this section of the book is unique within the exact definition of the word. Unique; and also intended to be positively beneficial for your health throughout all your remaining days. It deals with what's been missing in doctoring: *how to compensate for the bad effects of gravity on our health.* Compensate for these bad effects. Show you *what* the force of gravity is doing to destroy your health. And *how* this ceaseless down-thrusting force of gravity is ruining the functioning ability of various organs, making you older before your time, giving you mysterious aches and weaknessess you have not been able to get rid of, robbing you of your sexual vitality and so forth.

All of this would be pointless, however, if I did not also show you what you can do about it, and do it all by yourself for the most part, and benefit your health thereby.

Come, then. Let us consult together.

HOW TO RECOGNIZE THE COUNTER-GRAVITY AILMENTS

Because the human being is almost the only animal in the world that lives "against gravity," he alone suffers from what may be called *contra-gravity diseases.* Drooping eyelids; and they probably would not droop if they did not need to function so decidedly against gravity. Fallen stomach; and certainly there would not be this down-pull strain on the organ if it did not function straight up, entirely against gravity. Prolapsed uterus; an organ bearing up under unremitting counter-gravitational strain on its suspensory ligaments. Sagging colon; the poor lower bowel weighted down by just the digested food and food wastes in it, which would not be the case if it were horizontally positioned. Varicose veins; vessels full to bursting with blood needing to return to the heart but always having to make that straight uphill climb against gravity. Fallen arches; poor little seven bones that not only have to form the cantilever spring for the heavy body above, but also get the pounding of that weight with every step and mis-step, every fall and jar and jolting impact.

Why All This Happens to You

All this happens to you because you, as a human being, live unchangeably in a mechanically upright state. Performing bears and monkeys, it is true, walk on their hind legs from time to time. But they don't do it as a regular thing! You, however, always do your living and working in positions that oppose the force of gravity. Sitting, standing, walking, running, heaving, lugging, straining—all against gravity. Only during sleep do you customarily abandon your upright (counter-gravitational) stance. Any wonder that you have veins that bulge with blood, and a colon that's weighted down, and arches that fall—and all the rest?

Sure, our upright form of living has given us our civilization, and also the edge over other living creatures. But, everyone of us pays the price for it in imperfect health. For your existence against the force of gravity, you must *pay a toll* every livelong day of your life. With gravity steadily working against you, the ruinous effect in your case may show up in the diaphragm, the heart, the kidneys or other tissues that do not appear to have any connection with the contra-gravity diseases I have mentioned.

Nearly everyone I have ever examined has revealed a faulty diaphragm; faulty because it exists and functions against the force of gravity. Do you know what a poor diaphragm can mean? Breathing difficulties, for one thing. The inability to oxygenate properly and fully, for the diaphragm determines our ability to oxygenate or aerate the body and "burn up" the accumulated toxic waste products. In the animal the diaphragm is always in place, always so positioned that it can do its work well. In you and me, whether aware of it or not, the diaphragm and many organs besides, *pay the toll* in some way, and to some degree, because of needing to exist and work against the down-pulling force of gravity.

This is a toll for which we can compensate, however. Of course we pay a price for living against gravity, but I have discovered and developed a way to make up for the strains and stresses on our organism that we suffer because we exist in a straight uphill way, fighting the gravitational forces.

The animal does not have contra-gravity problems—no fallen

arches, for example—because its weight is distributed four ways, over four limbs. No diaphragm that has plopped out of position, for in the horizontal body this important organ does not undergird the lungs in constant defiance of gravity. No prolapsed uterus, or fallen stomach, or colon that has sagged to the point of resting on the pelvis, as is so often true in human beings.

YOU ARE AN UPSIDE-DOWN PYRAMID

Sara Blythe was only 18 but already an old woman in a lot of ways. She was flat-chested and breathed exclusively with the tips of her lungs. Her breaths were really short gasps, her eyes were lacking in spark. The poor thing had emphysema.

The first thing I did was ask her to get down on her hands and knees. In this position she could breathe more easily. It was because the diaphragm fell into place when she was thus placed. I had things to say to Sara, and said them while she was on hands and knees.

"Open your mouth and pant with your tummy," I told her. "Make that midriff of yours go in and out vigorously. Pant as you've seen a dog do. Every time you see that mid-section of yours go in and out, you're exercising the diaphragm. In your condition I want the diaphragm back in shape, and that'll put you back in shape."

As the girl continued working her diaphragmatic muscle (and thus strengthening it), I assured her that the power which created her can also heal her. Lest she think it's some kind of metaphysical philosophy I was preaching, I emphasized that this was a physical force. The body heals itself through a natural and quite marvelous *physical* force that can turn sickness into health in any part of the body. All it needs is a little guidance to direct this natural self-repairing power to the ailing organ. I could do the guiding, and I would. But Sara could also, for it was the kind of guidance I could teach her to apply to her own case for the benefit of her own health. This interested her enormously.

"Keep working that diaphragm," I counseled. She smiled at me and said she would. It was easier to do than she dreamed. When she tired of the Diaphragmatic Breathing I showed her how to do the Sway and Arch drill while still on hands and knees. "It's to give your vertebrae a chance to work themselves back where they belong, correcting the nerve pressure that blocks the transmission of Life Force to your chest area." When she sat up I did one Head Lift for her, then showed her that she could do it almost as easily all by herself. She knew that it was for the purpose of lifting nerve pressures in her neck that were interfering with the free flow of nerve impulses to the bronchi, lungs and diaphragm.

"Did you ever think that you are an upside-down pyramid?" I asked her. She never had. "You're an inverted pyramid actually," I explained. "One that is wide at the shoulders and tapers down to two tiny feet. You are forever balancing your entire weight on the space occupied by those two narrow feet. And it is so very easy to lose the structural balance of your body," I pointed out to her. "All the jars and jolts and falls and mis-steps you take. The way all that weight above pounds down on the vertebrae below. Almost everything from congested sinuses to fallen arches can be caused by your living against gravity in this way."

Sara said that this ought to have given doctors a clue to what's been missing in doctoring people. She was on to the Missing Link quite quickly. "Is that why you are having me do all this, Doctor?" she asked. "If animals do not suffer from a diaphragm in bad position, is that why you have me do these things in a horizontal position—to compensate for doing everything else against gravity?"

HOW TO ACHIEVE THE BENEFITS OF CORRECT OXYGENATION

The girl had touched on the main point—and the main organ. Living in opposition to the force of gravity causes many ills. She had cold extremities, especially cold toes, because the bloodflow from the ends of the circulation had to return to the heart straight uphill against gravity. She was constipated; and this was largely because foodstuffs piled up in the cecum, where the appendix lies, and had a cruel uphill climb to continue their digestive journey. But worst of all was the diaphragm, the organ which partitions the chest from the abdomen and the one upon which correct breathing absolutely depends. Breath, not bread, is the staff of life. To give her renewed life we had to give her a newly strengthened diaphragm.

The best way to reoxygenate the body, I've discovered, is to develop a strong working diaphragm, and her Diaphragmatic Breathing drills did that for Sara. Then I introduced her to Double Count Exhalations: inhaling to the count of four or six and exhaling to double that count. This was fun. It was more than that, for in developing these techniques I found that the very best way to strengthen our breathing apparatus is to exhale under control. Sara got it up to 8 and 16: inhaling to 8 and then exhaling *under control* until she came to 16. While rationing out the exhaled air until reaching that high count, she felt the midriff muscles working, developing, strengthening. I added the Dowager's Hump to her program (see *Glossary* for all these drills) and her flat chest came up and out, to her delight.

YOU HAVE TWO STRIKES AGAINST YOU

"Hey, these are wonderful!" Sara said to me one day in a burst of exuberance. She had come into the office after a long walk, counting her exhalations as she went. Now, out of the public eye, she did a few Dowager's Hump drills, and I'd just shown her the best of the lot, the Primordial Walk. This is perhaps the best single program for overcoming the effects of gravity on our health. Along with the Diaphragmatic Breathing which begins to oxygenate the system, one need look for little more by way of exercise if he does not have the time for more. "I'll bet," Sara continued as she did the Primordial Walk around my consulting room, "that what I'm doing is enough to make up for what you call 'the toll that we must pay for living against gravity.' "

"Sara," I said, "we just have to come to grips with reality in this matter. We have two strikes against us merely from the fact that we happen to live vertically instead of horizontally." This was her kind of language. Two strikes, huh?

"Yes. Number one is that we tend to become shorter in stature as we grow older, all because of the gravitational downhill drag on our body—on the discs between the vertebrae, actually. There is almost constant bodily weight on those little flexible discs, which never would occur if we were horizontal animals. Therefore, the discs get thinner with advancing years; but, fortunately, we've developed a way to decompress the discs that's almost a perfect counter-measure for the problem. That's number one. Number two is your trouble, meaning that we breathe poorly, and in a most shallow manner, because we live in an upright state that conduces toward inefficient breathing. When you were strong enough in your back muscles to lift yourself out of the baby crib that first time, that's when you began fighting gravity and began breathing with the apex of each lung rather than with the deeper lobes where the reserve air-power is stored. Only if you're a trained singer do you learn to use your diaphragm correctly. Or, maybe, if you're a long distance runner and hold out doggedly until you reach what is called 'second wind'—then you tap the residual air of your lung reserves."

Sara gave a bit of extra effort to her Primordial Walk and then stood up to do some vigorous Dowager's Hump drills while energetically panting the Diaphragmatic Breathing drill at the same time. "No two strikes against me, Doc! Not anymore, because I'm hep," she chirped gleefully. I remembered the little old lady of 18 with flat chest and tired eyes that I'd first seen only a few weeks before, and I knew that Sara Blythe was well. She certainly was, as she said, *hep.*

WHAT WE MUST UNDERSTAND AND DO ABOUT
VARICOSE VEINS AND RUPTURES

The fact of living "uprightly" often causes an excess of blood-weight on the valves of our veins. This is especially so when we strain with a downward pressure upon the legs and the floor of the abdomen. That's the beginning of varicose veins; also of hernias and other tears in muscle fibers of the body.

Helen Best was living proof of this. She was a stout lady of 40-odd years with chronic bronchial asthma and legs bulging with varicose veins. In the days of their beginnings, she and her husband had run a general store where she did lifting and heaving of barrels and cases because Mr. Best was a slight, scholarly man, not suited to business at all. Mrs. Best was on her feet 14 hours a day for years, and this was hardly interrupted when she had her babies. Thus her vein-valves ballooned and almost burst, her weight increased to her further disadvantage, and she wheezed so that you could hear her breathing across a room.

When I advised the lady to Run Backwards in a Pool every day and also oxygenate by way of Diaphragmatic Breathing, a new world of leg-ease began for her. But what will benefit the reader most is the unbelievable truth that virtually the same general health rules that helped the flat-chested, 18-year-old Sara Blythe with emphysema, miraculously tuned up and restored the stout, middle-aged Mrs. Best with asthma.

I trust the reader will note well what follows. *Asthma is easy to help.* The fact that asthmatics suffer without improvement only shows how much missing in doctoring is The Missing Link. In asthmatics, the diaphragm must be aided first. Once, I could hear the stout lady's labored "musical chest" breathing clear back in my consulting room from the waiting room. She was having an asthmatic attack, and her thin-shouldered husband was standing beside her, helplessly wringing his hands. All I did was stand behind the lady and embrace her middle area with both hands, then *lifted the entire tummy and diaphragm* upward, as though trying to push it up under the ribs and breastbone.

How to Stop an Asthma Attack
By Hugging the Victim

Almost at once, she heaved a sigh of relief, as she got rid of the breath that was trapped and couldn't get out. (People think asthmatics can't catch their breaths; the truth is they can't let out the breath they've got.) With Mrs. Best's breath returned, I marched her and her husband back to my examining room and told her to get down on hands and knees; whereupon I straddled her as though she were a little pony, reached my arms under tummy and lifted the whole mass of flesh toward her spine and up under her ribs. This put the diaphragm further into place and made her breathe as easily as a baby. "What's the matter with you, sir?" I charged at her husband. "Have you forgotten how to hug your wife anymore?" I had him embrace and lift her diaphragm from behind, both while she was standing and on hands and knees, and assured him that this technique would work because it was natural—nature's own way of putting the diaphragm back into position.

I repeat that asthma is almost always very easy to help. Several simple rules must be observed, then you are free of enslavement to adrenalin and other bronchial antispasmodics and general drugs.

1. Re-position the diaphragm by means of counter-gravitational drills such as the Knee-Chest, the Head-Hang, and the Primordial Walk. 2. Correct nerve pressures and normalize the vaso-dilators by means of the Dowager's Hump, the Sway and Arch, the Head Lift. 3. Oxygenate those bronchial tubes by means of Diaphragmatic Breathing and Double-Count Exhalations. 4. By all means keep mucus-forming foods from getting into that digestive tract. If the asthmatic does not have the needless load of caring for eggs, cheeses, butter, meat fats, salt, sugar and the rest (see *Glossary* and list of mucus-forming foods), it hardly matters how young or old he is—he can be helped, and will be, to a hardly imagined degree.

HOW TO VIEW FACIAL NEURALGIA

Thousands of people have feet with fallen arches and other sagging organs, conditions stemming from the gravitational down-pounding of bodily weight upon their various structural parts. Among the worst are trifacial neuralgias and tics and sagging facial tissues served by one or more of the cranial nerves. (See next page, "What to Do for Sagging Facial Muscles.") These ailments are not encountered in animals existing in the horizontal position.

Nearly all gravitational ailments can be helped or reversed if we but understand the facts of counter-gravitation, and if we choose to follow the Missing Link programs here presented.

Our doctors customarily aren't trained at all in contra-gravity diseases. They do not recognize them as such, and can do nothing about them. They do not in fact even examine for, or notice, such problems in their usual checkups. The consequence is that the ailments caused by the force of gravity go unattended, for certainly no pill or injection can reach a problem caused by the downward pull of gravity such as fallen arches, thinned intervertebral discs, a sagging colon, prolapsed uterus or badly functioning diaphragm.

HOW TO LISTEN TO THE WISDOM OF THE BODY

"O Lord," goes the prayer, "grant me the serenity to accept that which I cannot change, the power to change that which I can, and the wisdom to know the difference." With two strikes already against us—living against gravity, plus living in a polluted atmosphere—there is high wisdom in paying heed to what we *can* do something about. What, then, can we do? Specifically, we can follow the Missing Link program herein set forth which enables almost anyone to overcome the baneful effects of living against gravity. Also, we can at the same time as we do our counter-gravitational drills, achieve the high rewards of better oxygenation through a strengthening of the breathing apparatus, correction of nerve pressures almost anywhere in the body, purification of our bloodstreams through detoxifying the system and the proven easy ways of eliminating nervous tension from this hard-driving hurry-flurry existence.

Let us, therefore, *listen to the wisdom of the body.* Some things you can change, some you can't. As always in our Missing Link program, let's begin with the top and proceed downward.

WHAT TO DO FOR SAGGING FACIAL MUSCLES

Doctors are baffled by Bell's palsy, a kind of paralysis of the face first noted by a Scottish physiologist in the 18th century. Also trifacial neuralgia and tic douloureux and other conditions which involve a sagging of facial muscles and tissues. The shooting pains are suffered along the pathways and distributions of the cranial nerves that supply the face with *operating messages* and *functional power.*

These cases are usually without any evidence of organic change, and are for the most part untreatable. In all such cases, however, I long ago observed a curious and startling common denominator. The one thing that these cases had in common, I noticed, was a condition of pinched nerves in the neck. *There were no exceptions.* Dealing with several hundred cases of this kind, I found nerve-root compressions were discoverable in all of them.

How did I happen to run into this discovery? It was easy, really. All I did was ask the patients to turn their heads, first to one side and then to the other. They would turn as far as they could, *without jerking,* as though trying to reach the tip of the shoulder with the end of the chin. Normally, one should have equal mobility in both directions. But not one of these cases could turn as far to one side as to the other. This matter of unequal mobility of the neck was the one thing all of them had in common.

It became as clear as day that what was needed by all these patients with nerve compressions that interfered with the flow of Life Force to facial tissues was to *lift the pressures off the nerves.* It brought forth a new technique: the Head-Lift (see *Glossary*). It's one of the most important drills any sick person can do for himself, and it was born as the result of nerve pressures we observed in the necks of facial neuralgia cases.

TEST YOURSELF: CAN YOU TURN YOUR HEAD EQUALLY?

From my understanding of counter-gravity ailments I knew at once that it is *impossible to have unequal neck mobility without also having cervical nerve-root compressions.* This means that if you cannot turn your head as far one way as the other—turning all the way on both sides—you are suffering, without a doubt, some degree of pinched nerves somewhere in your neck. It cannot be otherwise. Test yourself. Ask another person to tell you if you can turn equally far in both directions, without jerking your head either to left or right (for often you cannot tell this by yourself). If you fail to turn as far one way as the other, then nerves to your facial tissues, or to the head, or even to any part of the body below, may be pinched and amenable to correction.

If the reader understands what is written here, he's made a vast forward stride toward understanding how to gain and maintain health. If the reader will also try to understand what follows in this section of the book, he will know what is at present unknown to many professionals in the various healing arts, doctors though they are. It concerns the human neck, as differentiated from the neck of the four-footed animal, and why our neck causes us so many exasperating, aggravating maladies.

WHAT YOU MUST KNOW TO SAVE YOUR NECK

Note this, please. Our neck is not protected by ribs. It is precariously balanced upright and curved, concavely, to maintain its balance. It cannot be forgotten that the human spine is structurally like the animal spine. The formation and operation of what the anatomists call pre- and post-zygapophyses of the vertebrae prove to the scholar that *we are constructed to function horizontally rather than vertically*. In the horizontal position the neck hangs *down*. No strain on it. The powerful, heavy neck muscles elongate as the animal grazes or merely walks along. The very heaviest of these (called sternocleidomastoids) serve as dependable strong protectors for the nerve lines within the neck. That is so when we're horizontally positioned. But when we lift ourselves up on our hind legs, well, we just have to curve our neck backward in order to balance the head aloft. The several layers of muscles which overlap the spinal bones of the neck pull in every-which-way direction as we twist and turn. The imbalance of these muscles pulls upon, and changes, the position of the neck vertebrae—and this *always* causes a state of pinched nerves.

To save our very necks, we must keep the nerve pathways free of pressures. Otherwise, being pinched, they cannot transmit the nerve impulses and directional messages that give energy and functional power to the organs served by such nerves. So we absolutely have to *lift the pressures* which we accumulate by our upright plan of living, lift them off the nerves, and in the following pages we give you specific techniques for doing exactly this, thus enabling you to compensate for the effects of living against gravity.

Get the idea, then all else follows. You will be well on your way with protective knowledge for good solid future health if you get the idea of how the neck works—or really *mis-works*—for then you will know how to do things to make up for the ill effects of counter-gravitational existence. Just remember that your head twists and turns *in an upward state,* not downward as it would if you were a horizontal structure. In that upward state, the neck muscles, working against gravity, shorten and contract, work against each other, pull against their attachments (at the collarbones and mastoids for example), and, acting very much like guy wires attached to a central pole, they shorten on one side and are pulled too long (overdrawn) on the other. This is why you cannot turn your head as far one way as the other. Got the idea?

If you want to add to this the daily jarrings and joltings that you sustain in the course of living activities, then you've got the whole picture. Since the neck is not protected by ribs as are the vertebrae below, in its upright, precariously balanced state we can understand why we have neck tensions and "cricks" which produce nerve-pressure symptoms and ailments.

Most of us know what a vertebra is, and that there are seven of them in the neck. Between every two of them there must pass, from the central switchboard which is the spinal cord, the individual nerves that supply all the various organs with different kinds of power. Whatever organ or tissue is at the end of any nerve line must receive through or over that nerve the *functional power* that it depends upon. Also its *directional power,* meaning the messages which tell it how to coordinate with the rest of the body. Also the *self-repairing energy* which enables the organ to repair its damaged cells, for the human organism can repair itself with its own manufactured ingredients, unlike a piece of wood or a hunk of iron that cannot fill in its nicks and holes when gouged or scratched. But—*note this well!*—the organ that depends on nerves for all this cannot be healthy if it is deprived of these various kinds of power because the nerves are pinched in the neck, unable to transmit the needed impulses.

You and I are today the end-result of all the strains and stresses of our lifetime. Since all the jarring impacts or bad falls we've had can cause those heavy muscles in our neck to shorten and lengthen like guy wires, the vertebrae are pulled out of position and pinch the nerves which transmit the vital functional, directional, healing power to organs.

HOW TO EVALUATE THE FACTS

I was teaching a class in London and invited the attending doctors of chiropractic, osteopathy and naturopathy to bring before the group any particularly difficult cases they were caring for, the idea being to make a neurological evaluation in front of the class for the benefit of all. The next morning one eminent Harley Street doctor came with a patient who'd had a "fixed torticollis" for many years—a kind of wry neck that enabled him to turn his head only one way. The man's head was grotesquely positioned over his left shoulder and he could not see to the right unless he turned his whole body. I pointed out to the class how very severe this Mr. Edgar Butler's nerve pressure was in the neck, then did a ridiculously simple lift that anyone could have done, and one which is given in the *Glossary* as the Head-Lift.

How to Deal with Wry Neck or Stiff Neck
Very Easily All By Yourself

By merely placing my open hands on his neck, just under the mastoid bones, and lifting and turning him further toward the left—his nerve pressures were released. It was a Head-Lift, exactly the same as given in chapter 12 of this book. But in this case it was done only toward the left side, for that was the side he could turn to, and *it does not accord with physiology to go against the strains of the body.* Going toward the right, the side to which Mr. Butler could not turn, would not be *listening to the wisdom of the body.* As I did the Lift, and turned his head toward the left as I lifted, the man's chronic torticollis left him and he was able to turn toward the right for the first time in years.

The reader already knows that I cannot abide any of the fanciful theories in doctoring that do not accord with physiology. Theories like that of giving lesser diseases (cowpox), through shots, in order to prevent greater diseases (smallpox) from invading the body; for, as already noted, the body has its natural selectivity which is violated when we push substances directly into the bloodstream, without first having them go through the digestive process. And, as already noted also, my own theory, which *does* accord with physiology, is that disease is perpetuated in human beings by shots which pollute bloodstreams and weaken resistance against disease.

In general doctoring, there is a theory that we must force bodily parts that function wrongly toward the direction that is correct. But this does not accord with physiology, and it does not listen to the body's own inner wisdom. In this simple technique for a wry neck or stiff neck, for example, you do the Head-Lift only to one side, the side toward which the ailing person can turn *with comfort.* Forcing it toward the other direction (just because it "ought to turn there") can be ruinous and cause tissue damage. Working "with the body" is the physiologically correct way.

The reader can probably see the inherent rightness and wisdom of the foregoing, but many doctors will not be able to go along because they have been trained in opposite directions. (In the Bible, the brilliant and scholarly Nicodemus could not understand what the less-trained villager with his "gutter wisdom" could understand at once.) It is because they do not understand these essentials that doctors have probably never examined you to determine if you can turn your head as far one way as you can the other way. Therefore, they have *missed* knowing whether the nerves in your neck are pinched or blocked, unable to transmit nerve impulses to organs below which are sick because they are deprived of such power impulses.

HOW YOU CAN TEST AND EXAMINE YOURSELF

Whether you have a trifacial neuralgia, headaches or eye pains or ear problems, you can quite adequately test yourself to learn if you are the victim of nerve pressures in the neck. *Go to a mirror and look at yourself with face straight front.* Are your earlobes even, or does one appear much lower than its mate? If the answer is yes, you may be unwittingly and automatically leaning your head away from where it hurts—where the nerve is pinched or irritated. If you have been going without relief to a doctor who's given you drugs or injections for that facial neuralgia or migraine condition, you may have the answer to his lack of results right there. No drug or injection can lift a vertebral pressure off a nerve, but with the Head-Lift and other techniques in the *Glossary* of this book you surely can.

Now observe your shoulders. Is one so much lower than the other that the tailor must put in a pad to make your two shoulders appear even? (This means that there is a lateral curvature already started or in process of forming in your upper spine, and how can a pill or shot possibly lift that low shoulder?) And look at the point of your chin: is it directly under your nose or off to one side? And if you own two bathroom scales, just stand with one foot on each of them, feet equidistantly apart. Do you weigh the same on both sides or several pounds more on one side? I can assure you now that being right- or left-handed has nothing to do with being heavier on one side or the other; it's due, probably, to a former fall or jarring impact that caused you to be jolted out of normal center of gravity, and in that case you are dragging to one side, suffering from an "energy leak" condition as you unawaredly try to fight yourself back into center, using up your energy to achieve nothing at all. Having tested and examined yourself in this way, you know that the doctors you've gone to haven't paid the scarcest attention to any of these important criteria; they've only given you pills and shots for mechanical stresses and strains that have thrown you out of adjustment. Ridiculous, isn't it? No wonder people go to a doctor for 20 years and are still sick, or sicker than they were when they started. They've been going to the wrong *kind* of doctor—one trained in pharmacology, not in mechanics of the body.

HOW TO TELL WHETHER YOU ARE
IN OR OUT OF HEALTHY MECHANICAL ADJUSTMENT

During many years of practice, I've so often heard the self-irritated remarks of patients who finally discovered the futility of taking drugs or injections for a body out of mechanical adjustment, due to living against gravity, and accumulating nerve pressures from their falls, jolts, and daily strains. A low shoulder; a head that cannot turn as far to the right as to the left; an earlobe that's much lower than its opposite; a chin that's not directly under the nose but off to the right or left of it; a short leg, or curvature, or high hip. "Why," they declare with self-disgust at being taken in by allopathic doctors who gave them drugs to cure nerve pressures, "how could I have been so stupid! It was as illogical as going to an occulist for your teeth or to a dentist for new eyeglasses!"

You can tell quite easily if you are out of adjustment, merely by testing yourself in front of a mirror, as advised before. If you find that you actually are out of adjustment, and most people are to some degree, considering the counter-gravitational way we live and strain, you need the programs given in this book as you need the breath of life. All too often, the regular allopaths who know nothing about the mechanical ill effects on the body will pooh-pooh the very idea of leaving them for other doctors—so don't ask them. How often the allopaths scorn and even deprecate all doctoring sciences other than their own! It's a sure sign, of course, that they simply know nothing about other healing arts and are irritated by the presence of competitive methods. People in all classes are down on what they're not up on.

HOW TO FIND OUT IF YOU ARE
"LEAKING" ENERGY NEEDLESSLY

Do you own a plain carpenter's plumb line? If you do, hang it from the ceiling and stand in front of it. It will further astonish you, for it's a test of being out of adjustment that can hardly be improved upon. (Try testing a loved one with it.) Place your two feet exactly where the plumb bob at the bottom is between your ankles. Standing like this, you would naturally expect the plumb line to go upward between the knees, genitals, pubic bone, navel, breastbone and center of forehead. That is how it would bisect your body—split it in even halves—if you were in adjustment mechanically.

In most cases, however, what you will see as you follow the plumb line upward with your eye will rock you. The line begins between your ankles all right, but from there it usually wanders off so far to the left or right that it crosses your chest like a diagonal sash instead of a medial line.

This means that you are being gravitationally *pulled* out of center. Throughout the day, there's a constant "leak" of energy as you try to work your offside-pulling body back into center. You are not aware of this, of course. Like every machine, you have a center of gravity—I call it in classes with doctors "our COG." As the result of a fall or jarring impact, this center of gravity of yours (COG) has somehow been yanked out of its proper mechanical position. If the ascending plumb line is seen cutting through your shoulder, for example, instead of through the exact middle of your forehead, you have proof of a force pulling you out of center with terrific power. You are dragging to the side, *leaking energy*. Like a car that's been in a severe collision and thereafter drags to one side, you've sustained in your life some kind of jolts or falls that have thrown your COG out of whack. Daily and hourly thereafter, you are endeavoring to fight yourself back into balanced center, expending energy thereby.

HAVE YOU JOLTED YOUR CENTER OF GRAVITY OUT OF POSITION?

Mrs. Flora Greeley was in good health, she said, but merely tired. The social whirl she was in required energy, and her lack of pep was a matter of deep concern. The two bathroom scales showed her 15 pounds heavier on one side. An osteopath she had gone to had discovered what he called "a short leg" and advised a heel lift to be placed on the shoe of her bad, short side. This I could not go along with, for my researches had proved to me beyond reasonable doubt that it was contrary to physiology. What the heel lift on the shoe of the short leg did was permanize the trouble and cure nothing. As I ask in my classes sometimes: How do you know that it is a short leg; what makes you sure the other isn't a long leg? I advise the doctors in my seminars to avoid the use of heel lifts because there is rarely a real anatomical, congenital short leg—only a *seeming* difference in leg lengths. Usually the head of the thigh-bone is found to have been turned or strained out of its socket, and when rotated into normal position the legs that seemed uneven are exactly similar in length.

Anyway, our socialite lady was way offside on the plumb line and weighed much heavier on the right when tested on two scales.

How to Stretch Yourself
Out of a Curvature

Discovering that she was a bowler, golfer, and tennis buff, I prohibited every one of these sports. Why did I do this? Because they are unilateral exercises. They are one-sided; and what this already-offside patient needed was a program to equalize *both* sides of her body. She grumbled, but when I explained that this was only for a while, until she was mechanically right, she agreed to discontinue the unilateral activities. I advised her to stretch against the wall. Standing with her short side touching the wall, she was to reach upward as high as she could, *without raising her heels,* and touch the wall, reaching a bit higher every day. This was in accord with physiology. I was obeying the wisdom of the body. I also advised that she do this most especially at bedtime, for what she gained at that hour she took to bed with her for metabolic profits of self-healing all through the night—and this accorded with physiology.

When I gave this high-toned lady the Primordial Walk, that was the limit. She yelped like a stuck pig, saying it was unladylike and immodest and ungraceful and worse. But soon she had her entire group of staid dowagers doing the same ungraceful drill and loving it. For them it was a prank—and it was fun. They all did the Sway and Arch and the Head-Lift also. It soon got to be evident that as soon as I instructed Mrs. Greeley in anything the whole country club set of hers had it the next day.

This became a real peril, for in time they swooped down on me for personal service, and for a while I was a kind of first-name-calling-society doctor against my desire. But the fact to report is this. The lady who first came because she lacked energy soon brought her offside body into mechanical adjustment and had energy to spare. Together with her ladies, she whooped it up as she hadn't done since boarding school. All the ladies even went beyond my instructions and refused to swim in any way but the breast stroke and Australian crawl. "The side stroke is offside and does not accord with physiology," one social arbiter told me with a straight face. "Oh, that is true," I replied, and thanked her with equal gravity.

When I researched the center of gravity factor some years ago, and began teaching its associated corrective techniques in doctor-seminars around the country, we had a saying that I advised the attending doctors to recite in class. "Restore the COG and you restore the patient." By thus repeating this saying they would "remember to remember" the large salient truth of this. It was far more than a catchphrase. When the knowledgeable doctor finds you out of gravity-center and brings you back to your in-center position, he almost always, at the same time, restores to you great energy reserves that you've been squandering in fighting the off-center pulls on your body. Nothing to take by way of medicine to achieve this. Just compensate for the gravitational ills and the body cures itself with its own, dependable, ever-present *Health Power.*

ANOTHER TEST YOU SHOULD MAKE THAT'LL SURPRISE YOU

You already know how to test yourself to some extent and determine whether you are in proper adjustment as a working machine. Now, to make assurance doubly sure, stand at the *side* of your plumb line and have a look. Instead of facing it with the plumb bob at the bottom between your ankles, now stand alongside the line so that the bottom of it touches the point of your ankle.

Another surprise awaits you. You would naturally expect the plumb line to go upward from where it starts at your ankle, go straight upward and cut through the middle of your knee, the center of your hip-bone, the point of your shoulder, the exact tragus (little protruding cartilage) of your ear, and so on. But does it? Not usually. I have examined thousands with this test and can tell you flatly that *nearly everyone leans forward of the string.* With the plumb line at the tip of the ankle bone, looking at the patient from the side, the rest of the body above the feet leans, and even sways, progressively forward—as though a hidden force is dragging or pushing it forward toward the front.

Here again, without being in the least aware of it, the majority of people are expending energy constantly. They are "leaking" energy reserves just to keep from falling forward on their faces. It's as though the entire pelvic bowl upon which the remainder of the body rests has been tipped forward: as though someone pushed the tops of both hips forward and pulled the bottom of the pelvic bowl (coccyx) backward. Can you see what this causes? The entire upper part of you rests upon nothing, so to speak, instead of resting solidly upon a pelvic platform that should support it like a solid cross-beam.

Now you can understand at once why so many of us suffer from what is called "sway-back." In the next chapter, and in the *Glossary* of chapter 12, I've described the Pelvic Back-Tip which is a perfect corrective drill for the sway-backed, hollowed-out lower spine. Right here, however, I hope to make sure that you understand utterly and completely that you really are out of mechanical adjustment *as a machine.* That besides being a chemical factory you are a machine, one which can and does get out of order and causes definite ailments. That your way of *living against gravity* makes it almost impossible not to be out of mechanical whack from time to time. That most of your, and your friends' so-called "incurable" ailments, are caused by the bodily machine being mechanically out of kilter, which in turn causes nerve pressures that interfere with the flow of functional energy to the various organs.

These matters relate to mechanical, counter-gravitational causes of disease. Yet they are matters which our doctors have not noticed, or studied, or done anything about. Until you learn to *compensate for living against gravity* and get that ailing body of yours hooked into a correct center of gravity, however, you will suffer from nerve pressures which prevent delivery, to the ailing organs, of the self-healing elements required for a miracle tune-up and rejuvenated health.

WHAT WE OUGHT TO KNOW ABOUT "SUBLUXATIONS"

From time to time we become definitely aware that we are mechanically askew and need mechanical correction of some kind. We often get diverted from this, however. In our profit-motivated society there's always a rush to sell us this-and-that "new" medicine or "just discovered" treatment of great promise. So we get side-tracked from the mechanical corrective measures that we need, since there are no salesmen pushing them at us. But now and then there's an item in the press or radio that makes us feel guilty (or stupid) about not attending to the body's demonstrable needs.

Doctors of chiropractic refer to the "subluxations" that our daily falls and jolts and strains and stresses cause to form in the human spine. The medical people complained that there were no such things; that this was a mere figment of the chiropractic imagination. Thus does one healing profession take umbrage at what another healing profession advances—an impossible, uncivilized situation that's further evidence of the profit motive. But occasionally we run into a smallish mention of this "subluxation" business in the medical press, and this straightens us out as to where the truth really lies.

In the *Journal of the A.M.A.* (Vol. 104) there appeared a little item that should direct us to the need of mechanical corrections. "Since the first of the year," said the item, "there have been 66 cases of unilateral subluxation of the cervical vertebrae without associated fracture seen in the fracture service of the Presbyterian

Hospital. . . . This sudden and spectacular increase [in subluxations] is not due to any change in the neck structure of New York's population but to the *education of the staff* in recognition of the condition." (Italics are mine.)

A subluxation is a condition of nerve pressure that exists because a vertebra of the spine has been jolted or strained out of its correct position. It is less than a "luxation," which means less than a dislocation; it's just enough *out of place* to make smaller or narrower the window in the bones through which the nerves must pass. It occurs frequently; it has occurred in you; hardly anyone fails to accumulate nerve-pinching subluxations as the result of living and straining against gravity. This sounds frightening, and in a way it is. But it needn't be now, for in this book you have specific drills and programs by which you can mend and correct nearly all the subluxations in your body as they occur—and those impossible of self-correction the trained doctor of chiropractic can attend to for you. At least, he can give you the start, after which you can complete the corrections, and prevent new ones, by means of the Head-Lift and Dowager's Hump, the Neck Traction and Sway and Arch, the Squat Drill and very important Pelvic Back-Tip.

What we ought to know about these ubiquitous, universally-occurring and frequently-met subluxations is, first, that they can be corrected, usually all by yourself by means of the drills set forth in the *Glossary* of chapter 12, and, secondly, that taking drugs or injections for subluxations is as useful as howling at the wind to stop blowing. Unfortunately, despite the evidence and recognition of subluxations as one of the truly major causes of human disease (especially the way the human is counter-gravitationally poised), now, as of yore, many doctors prescribe drugs and sera and intra-muscular shots—just as though injectibles can reshape the body mechanically!

HAVE YOU EVER HAD A "CRICK" IN THE NECK?

Esther Bromley had what she called a "kink" in her neck. She said her family described it as a "crick," as though it were something funny. But it wasn't a simple or a *nothing* item. One eye pained severely. She had a continuing headache. She was dizzy. Her temple throbbed. She'd been given a bedside-stand full of drugs. Nothing.

I had her throw out all the drugs and corrected the "crick" in a moment, then showed her how to do it herself. Hardly anything to it. But Esther was no fool. "Nothing to getting a scary, darkened room all bright and cheerfully lighted just by pushing a button," she said. "But, oh burrrother! If you don't know where's the button." It was exactly true. I'd spent a lot of silly years researching the human neck before I found that simple Head-Lift that anyone can be taught to do so easily. (See *Glossary.*) On mentioning this to a brilliant physicist who came to the office, I got a perfect parallel answer. "Edison spent years and did over 600 experiments just to find that filament that makes incandescent lighting possible," he said. "But we—by just a fractional second of pushing a button or pulling a light chain—can make all his hard efforts work for us in a jiffy, easy as pie."

The little item from a famous medical journal, which I quoted above, was what I now showed Esther Bromley. It concluded with a statement of *how* subluxations got started in human beings—how those nerve pressures which devitalized and debilitated and destroyed health actually were caused. Note, please.

> The initiating trauma is apt to be *very slight* but to occur when the muscles are off guard, as for example when the patient has just awakened. A sudden *kink* on stretching in bed, a *turn* in answer to a call, a *jerk of the head* to catch a forward pass, *a twist in taking off a dress* over the head, has been cited as the *cause* for the symptoms from which the patient sought relief. (Italics are mine.)

"That's it!" Esther cried. "A twist in taking off a dress, that's what I did. Imagine all that trouble coming from just such a common, everyday thing! (If she only knew how the force of counter-gravitational living was against her in this simple effort!) And imagine the nut I was," she continued, "taking all those pills to correct something caused by a vertebra in the neck out of place!"

WHAT YOU MUST KNOW ABOUT YOUR
NERVOUS SYSTEM FOR BETTER HEALTH

Now we begin to see why we are a nation of un-cured people, with almost every major disease known to man increasing rather than decreasing. More heart disease, cancer, mental illness, Parkinson's disease, epilepsy, cerebral palsy, diabetes, arthritis, muscular dystrophy, multiple sclerosis—where does the list end?

Our doctors know, or are supposed to know (considering the astronomical fees charged by them), that it's the nerves which supply all functioning parts of the body with power. It's the nerves that deliver to the various organs the power to do their work, the power to coordinate their functions and activities with the rest of the body, the power to heal and repair their own tissues damages. What you must know about the nervous system is that it is the body's Master System—and it is time that the doctors knew this too, and acted accordingly—not by giving drugs and injections to lift bony pressures off nerves, for instance!

It is known that the Master System of the body, which is our nervous system, is the *chief* to which all other systems are subordinate. All take their directions from the nervous system: your digestive system, respiratory system, cardio-vascular system, genito-urinary system and all the rest take their working and self-healing directions from your nervous system. Even the doctor who gave you a drug for subluxations studied this fact, only he forgot to act in accordance with it. It is too easy (or is it merely too profitable?) to prescribe a drug: "take some aspirins and rest in bed"—instead of learning *and doing* the techniques of lifting pressures off nerves.

**Does Your Body Exhibit These
Common Mechanical Faults?**

We must come to grips with the realities behind the ever-growing incidence of diseases listed above. Until doctors consider the terrible ill-effects of counter-gravity living on our health, *and learn to do something about it,* we cannot reasonably expect a downturn in our rising diseases. The average person weighs more on one side of his body than on the other. He cannot turn his head as far in one direction as the other. One shoulder is low, one hip high, one shoulder blade sticks out farther than its mate, one leg may be short (or long) relative to the normal one. If he stands before a plumb line he is seen shifting to the side; if you look at him from the side you see his poor "energy leaking" body leaning forward of the line, as though pushed there by an invisible force. All this is evidence to anyone—much less to one calling himself a doctor—that we are mechanically out of adjustment; and nobody but a fool expects a machine that is out of adjustment to be able to work (function) normally.

**Important Discovery: Your Pelvis
Can Slip Down in Front**

In the same frame of reference, we can tell you now (and take it up more fully later) about a most astonishing thing we have discovered. It is that many backaches that resist getting well, especially the stubborn and seemingly irremediable backaches of the lower spine, are due to something not hitherto known: namely, that the entire pelvic bowl slips in front. Slips downward. Gets pounded floorward by the pull of gravity, and must be put back, where it belongs mechanically, by applying an upward corrective technique. My research pinpointed this trouble of the spine and pelvis at one important spot where the initiating weakness occurs. For nearly eight years now, I have been teaching the doctors of chiropractic attending my seminars this vital new technique. At first, they were astounded to learn that, because we are constantly pounded down by gravity, human backaches and lumbosacral weaknesses do not come entirely from spinal problems in the spinal column itself, but also from slippage at that spot (tendon of Gracilis) just below the pubic bone in front.

This important discovery—that your pelvis can slip downward in front and cause back trouble not correctible by presently known techniques—is more fully set forth in the following chapter because you, the reader, can partly, if not wholly, *correct such slippage all by yourself if shown how.*

All other mechanical faults that your body can get into, *and does,* all that have been mentioned in this chapter will be taken up in the next chapter and you will be shown how to correct your own nerve-pinching mechanical problems—since most doctors don't know how to (or won't) do so.

CHAPTER TEN

How to Get Health Benefits
by Counteracting Destructive Effects
of Gravity--Specific Techniques

The reader has been left standing before a mirror (page 173) to test himself for mechanical faults, nerve pressures, bodily distortions, curvatures, and other signs of being out of adjustment. Now, in this chapter, he will be shown how to feel better immediately by applying the Missing Link counter-gravity programs.

This is the chapter for specific techniques and drills and programs. It is the place where I mean to show you what you can do to help yourself in all areas of health and how to do it.

Are you ready?

HOW TO GET RID OF PINCHED NERVES
IN THE NECK

Let's get back to that mirror as mentioned before. Let us discover once again which is your better side, the freer side of your neck, the side that has not accumulated nerve pressures or blockages. Facing the mirror, turn as far as you can toward the right. Just turn your head toward the tip of your right shoulder, without jerking or straining it. To be sure that you know how far you can turn, establish a fixed point out of the corner of your eye; that is, find a spot as far to the right as you can see during the turn, and that's your "fix." *It serves as your constant.* Now turn to the left as far as possible and fix your eye on a constant, as far to the left as you can see, probably a constant point on the wall behind your left shoulder.

Now you know which is your freer side, and which is the side to which you can turn the lesser distance. Thus you know where you want to release some of those nerve pressures in your neck. It'll be especially on the side where you can turn less.

Raise your elbows in front of you so your arms are parallel with the floor and fold the forearms backward until the palms touch the sides of your jaws. With open palms and fingers under the jaw-bones and around the curve of the neck, lift straight upward. Your palms will be hooked under the jawbones, and your open fingers as they extend backward will hook under the mastoid bones. With this as a kind of anchor, lift the head upward. *Lift the head off the neck and shoulders* in a straight upward line.

Do not curve the neck backward as you lift. The lift is exactly straight up; if anything, a bit forward of straight up. Do not press inward on the neck as you lift, for this may pinch the carotids or jugular veins and be suffocatingly unpleasant. The power and vigor of the lift is upward, not inward on the neck.

Now, as you lift the head vigorously upward, turn the face at the same time toward the right. Turn as far as you can, as far as your limit of motion will permit. Then, having turned to your limit of motion, give the head a little extra stretch. Not a jerking motion farther to the right, but just a bit of extra stretch beyond the ordinary limit of your turn. Do this several times. The tendency while turning the head is to slacken the lift, so *keep on lifting the head off the neck while turning it.* If possible, keep on lifting the head harder off the neck as you turn it. When you've come as far as you can turn, keep on lifting the head and try to stretch a bit beyond your limit of turning ability.

After doing this a few times, bend forward from the waist and do the same thing. Being bent forward from the waist, you now lift the head off the neck by pushing the head straight away—or forward—from the shoulders instead of straight upward. As before, turn to the right as you do this.

After having done this several times, a big, welcome surprise awaits you. Standing (or sitting) in the same position as when you first made a "fix" to determine how far you could turn, now turn your head to its limit without lifting it. Note the point of your "fix" on the wall behind your right shoulder. Wow! You can now see the wall behind you considerably farther and beyond the point of your original "fix." You have released the strain on your neck. You have *reversed the down-pull of gravity* on the vertebrae of your neck.

HOW YOUR HEALTH IS REJUVENATED BY THE
HEAD-LIFT TECHNIQUE

You have lifted the compression off the cervical vertebrae all by yourself. By this simple technique you have taken away at least *some* of the occluding, pinching, interfering pressure from the nerves of the neck. These nerves, now free of at least some of the pressure they suffered a moment ago, are at present able to transmit the nerve impulses to the organs they serve. They can now deliver to heretofore *deprived* facial areas (eyes, ears, nose, throat, sinuses, thyroid, besides scalp and arms and even the body below) the required nerve impulses and messages which direct their function, which coordinate their activities with the rest of the body, and which supervise the self-repair operations of the tissue cells.

Let's say that you can now see merely one inch farther on the wall behind your right shoulder than you could before you did this Head-Lift. Usually, the gain is considerably greater; but even if your gain was only an inch of mobility, then you have given yourself with this Head-Lift drill a full inch of free neck area that was formerly blocked. In this inch is where the interior down-traversing nerves and blood pathways had been pinched off and are now free. Free to transmit their products and messages and impulses down to organs and tissues of the body which had heretofore been *deprived.*

Having done the Head-Lift drill to the right, repeat it to the left. Take a "fix" on the wall behind your left shoulder and then, after doing the Head-Lift straight up, and also while leaning forward from the waist, take another "fix." Enjoy the delight of seeing how much farther you can now turn to the left. Again you have counter-gravitationally opened the nerve pathways and blood supply routes to the face and neck and other bodily areas. *Note:* The side to which you can turn less is the side which needs the Head-Lift most, so devote your efforts there.

TECHNIQUE FOR A BETTER FLOW
OF POWER TO YOUR BODY ORGANS

The foregoing Head-Lift drill is intended as a *specific* aid for such conditions as trifacial neuralgia, hearing malfunctions, facial rash, numbness of the tongue, and so forth. The fifth cranial nerve (trigeminus) which needs help here is also the nerve that transmits functional impulses and messages to the tongue and teeth and skin of the face; and it even branches off to the upper and lower jaws and hooks into the opthalmic nerve of the eye. Thus you can see how far-reaching this one simple technique can be in providing health benefits in various ailments. By giving yourself a workout with vigorous Head-Lift drills, you are compensating for the gravity strain on your delicate neck area, and should do this even if you have no ailments—just as a protective measure of incalculable value. But if you specifically need an improved flow of power and self-repairing impulses to any part of your face and neck, this is a major prescription in your case.

Besides the trifacial neuralgia and other conditions listed above, the Head-Lift is specifically recommended for drooping eyelids, eye tics and eyes that tear uncontrollably, spasms of the cheeks, headaches of almost any kind including migraines not amenable to other treatment, and almost any other affliction of the face and head—knowing for certain that if it does not quite help everything (for not all conditions are reversible), it will at least do general good by improving the nerve supply and be useful systemically.

WHY YOU SHOULD USE THIS TECHNIQUE ESPECIALLY AT BEDTIME

Mrs. G.J. Gayle came into the office with a facial spasm. From across the room anyone could see the flesh under her left eye "jump" erratically. It disturbed the lady greatly; and it appeared that in addition to the general drills for compensating against gravity-living, the Head-Lift was the *specific* aid she needed in her case.

She was taught to do the Head-Lift drill on her own after I did it for her that first time. My instructions were that she use this technique morning and night, but with especial vigor at bedtime. In those early days, I had not yet fully researched the Head-Lift drill and did not know its full value as an all-day technique, thinking it might be overdone. But the lady proved herself smarter than I was. (Doctors learn so very, very much from their patients, did you know this?) She began doing the Head-Lift all day long.

By using the technique on her own many times throughout the day, Mrs. Gayle observed some things worth reporting. When she felt a jumping spasm of her cheek coming on, she reported, she would hurriedly lift the head off the neck and shoulders, and this appeared to stop the spasm from starting. Sometimes it worked only moderately when she lifted the head straight up from a standing position; but, she said, on doing the Head-Lift with lots of force in the lift and turn *while bent from the waist,* the spasm would just barely try to start and then be aborted completely. Eventually, with the spasms caught before they began, they ceased altogether. It proved the usefulness of doing the Head-Lift as frequently as desired during the day.

I'd explained to the lady that the best and most useful time to do this drill was just before retiring. She wanted to know the reason for this. It was because, I explained, "at bedtime your weight will soon be off your feet, you'll no longer be fighting gravity for the next six or eight hours. The weight of your head and gravitational down-pull will not be pounding down on those neck vertebrae which compress the facial nerves while you're lying horizontally in bed."

This is true of all programs and exercises, as will be explained in this book from time to time because it is so important. Nowhere else in books by doctors do I see this vital advice given, yet the patient derives far greater value from self-help drills and programs at bedtime and should be told why. To digress for a moment, consider the value of the Diaphragmatic Breathing drill. If just before retiring, you go to your back yard or other place where the air is freshest and reoxygenate your lungs with this technique, all night long your system will have the advantage of that change-over of oxygen you've given it. The repair of your damaged and outworn tissue cells does not take place during your hyper-active day but during the quietude of the night. It is then that metabolic processes take over undisturbed, the breathing becomes slower and more rhythmic, and your heightened oxygenating capacity, as the result of Diaphragmatic Breathing, enables the body to repair itself better.

To derive greatest benefit from the Head-Lift, it should be done with especially vigorous lifting power at bedtime. Freeing the nerve pressures by lifting vertebral compressions at bedtime assures maximum gain from the drill all through the night.

TECHNIQUE FOR NERVOUS SPASMS OF THE FACE

The Head-Lift, as given above, is specifically intended for the conditions enumerated above.. But it is not the only natural self-aid for reaching facial conditions. Here is another counter-gravity measure that many have found to be extraordinarily helpful in what is called "tic douloureux."

Tic or Spasm of the Face. Place both open hands upon your face, fingers slightly overlapping, and do several rapid, very vigorous upsweeps on the facial skin. The hands are in tight contact with the chin at the start, then they sweep up rapidly from there to the forehead and around the scalp, lifting the skin and flesh of the face as they move from chin to scalp. Do this about a dozen times. Do it sitting up or even when lying down. This technique is *not* for bedtime; it is too stimulating and tends to keep one awake. (On rising in the morning, however, this Upsweep drill is a fine arouser and stimulator.)

TECHNIQUE FOR DROOPING LIPS AND MOUTH CORNERS

And here's another program that very often reaches a problem which bothers many persons, especially women. In this one we seek to strengthen and give tone to a muscle of the mouth. It's a muscle very much like a thick rubber band (*obicularis oris*) and has the function of wrinkling the lips and closing the entire mouth. Think of a rubber band that has lost its elasticity. Now imagine this band encircling your mouth and needing more "snap" in it, more of what physiologists call muscle tonicity.

With this in mind, hook your forefingers inside the corners of your lips. Imagining your fingers hooked into a rubber band, pull outward on a horizontal plane. Pull the lips apart, then at once let them snap back by releasing your fingerhold. Do this a dozen times or more; with every pull-out and snap-back you're giving more snap and tone to that mouth muscle that's like a rubber band.

Are you worried that this may spoil the contours of your mouth? That it may produce in you a *big mouth?* In this connection I recall the tongue-in-cheek drubbing handed me by Milady Hays.

"With all those horrid lines at the corners of my mouth," said Milady Hays, "I thought you were cruel to give me this rubberband-snapping folderol. It would give me such a big mouth, you will remember my saying to you. But when you vowed it would restore tone to the lip tissues and give me a small mouth instead of a big one, I followed your advice kind of reluctantly." She leaned forward conspiratorially. "Now I know it's true. Not only doesn't my mouth droop hardly (sic!) at all, but even the lines at the corner of my mouth are gone. It's great!"

HOW TO DECONGEST YOUR SINUSES

This quite wonderful self-help technique refers to the maxillary sinuses, the ones people usually talk about when they say "I have sinus trouble." These cavities, one on each side, fill up with debris or hardened mucus and give rise to severe pain. A common technique employed by the specialist to give temporary relief is that of forcing an object (needle or tube) through the large "hallway" in the upper jawbone. The idea is to unplug this hallway (antrum of Highmore) and allow its congestive wastes to drain off. My way, I believe without any doubt at all, is far better; besides which it does not hurt and does not cost a doctor's fee.

Touch the projection of your cheekbone with your thumb, one on each side. Now slide each thumb under the cheekbone and the bony shelf that you find there. Lift straight up with the fleshy part of your thumb. As you lift from under these bony shelves, slide your thumbs inward toward the middle of the face. When your thumbs are stopped at the juncture of the nose and cheek, give a little extra lift. This spot, where the nose and cheekbones join, will hurt a bit at times as you lift. Often you will hear a slight click as you lift. Immediately after the lift you will find, upon sniffing, that the nasal passages have cleared. Breathing is easy. Sinus congestion is gone. The results are as good as those you get from the specialist who pushes the needle through the hallway of the bone.

TECHNIQUE FOR WRINKLED SKIN
OF THE NECK

In middle-age there are three areas of the human body that usually break down ahead of other bodily tissues. One area is at the mouth; and we have already given a perfect exercise or "tonicity springback drill" named Technique for Drooping Lips and Mouth Corners. A second is the flesh of the upper arm known as the triceps; and I'll outline a technique for that sagging tissue that's adjacent to the armpit. Third is this neck muscle (the platysma myoides) which, like a thin neck-protector worn by the lancing knights of yore, covers all the front of you from the collarbones way up to the jawbone and cheeks and mouth.

In middle-age years, this very thin skin-like membrane tends to wrinkle and sag. It's a certain sign of what living against gravity does to us. The sagging process often begins at around the age of 40 (what Victor Hugo called the "old age of youth"), and unless we counteract the effects of gravity in some way, the wrinkling process continues rapidly.

The technique for "de-wrinkling" and "de-sagging" the skin of your neck is as follows. Lie on your back with the head hanging over the edge of the bed. Thus the head is lower than the body, face upward. In this position, do the "goldfish" drill. This means opening your mouth and closing it merely by *lifting the lower jaw up toward the upper jaw.* It's something like the workings of the mouth of a goldfish. This stretches the platysma muscle and unwrinkles the skin. Do it until tired.

A further aid is to sit and do a rapid pronouncing drill. Our letters "U" and "X" are pronounced in Spanish, phonetically, "Oooh" and "Eckus." I want you to say "Oooh" and Eckus" aloud and with energy, over and over again. As you do this, place the back of your hand up against the lower jaw and note the tightening and working of the skin and flesh. It will convince you of the powerful stimulus you are giving the sagging neck area.

HOW TO HELP SAGGING UPPER-ARM FLESH

Here we are going to deal with a kind of three-pronged muscle of the upper arm, just below the armpit. When it begins to sag in middle age, it's immediately noticeable and unsightly. The way to firm up this muscle is quite specific.

Raise your arms all the way up, as though reaching for the sky. Now, while being sure to hold the elbows there, drop the *forearms* straight back. Do not lower the elbows while doing this. That's the trick. The forearms hinge backward from the elbows; it's sometimes called "the hinge drill" for that reason. To repeat: arms straight up; elbows stay straight up; forearms only drop (hinge) backward, with your hands coming down to almost touch the back of your head while the elbows remain high. Do this until tired, especially at night. You will feel the effects of this workout precisely in those sagging triceps of the arms.

Another thing worth knowing is this. To bring firmness to this sagging muscle, you must push objects or weights away from you, not toward you. When exerting any effort toward you, as when raising a barbell toward your chest or when chinning yourself, you use the biceps rather than the triceps. When doing push-ups, however, the weight of the body is being forced away from you and the triceps are at work. In our usual activities we do not use the triceps very much: that's why they sag. The rule in life is: *What you don't use, you lose.* Nature takes away those functions which we do not employ. It is an absolute physiological rule. Remember that it applies to everything. Try to use all your functions and capabilities until the last day of your life: memory, sex, singing and speech, bodily movements, everything. What you do not use you lose.

WHAT TO DO FOR ROUND SHOULDERS
AND A HUNCHED SPINE

One very noticeable way that we pay the toll for living against gravity is the stooped upper back that many people acquire. The upper spine tends to stoop into what is called a kyphosis, or curvature, from the years and effort of sustaining our weight upward, against the force of gravity. Women are especially aware of this and refer to it as "Dowager's Hump," the same name that I've given one of the important drills for restoring structural integrity to the spine and releasing nerve pressures from the upper vertebrae.

Do you remember the test in the previous chapter (page 174) which revealed that when standing beside a plumb line nearly everyone is shown to lean forward at the shoulders? Instead of standing straight up, most of us are forward of the central line at the upper spine. The toll that is exacted from us for existing in defiance of gravity often begins right there—with a stooped, round-shouldered condition. Fortunately, we have a quite perfect drill to compensate for this.

Clasp your hands behind your back, both palms open and touching. With palms contacting each other in back of you, roll the elbows *inward*. Try to make the elbows actually touch each other. As you do this, look at yourself in a mirror from the side. Note that the upper vertebrae of the spine straighten out of the humped, stooped state. Note also that you stand taller. And that your chest pushes forward, exercising the pectoral muscles and inducing better chest development.

I recall the case of young Joanie King, a teenager who had a spindly body and quite lethargic disposition. Her shoulders stooped and seemed to droop into a flat, hollow chest. She seemed to take no great interest in anything, was always tired and uncaring about passing events.

It wasn't until I mentioned the term "Dowager's Hump" that Joanie showed interest. It appears that she had read something about it, and the story I told her confirmed it. It was about the young lady who had served as the model for Miss Liberty on our quarters and half dollars. This was a true story of an emaciated girl in her late teens whose idol was Annette Kellerman, a beautifully-formed swimming champion of that day. To attain the bodily proportions of her idol, the emaciated girl began doing the above-mentioned exercise for round shoulders, doing it all day until nearly exhausted.

With this one exercise alone, the thin young lady developed a full chest and straight body and such an excellent figure that she could serve as the model for Miss Liberty on our coins.

What Miss Liberty could do, Joanie decided that she could do. And it worked. She did the Dowager's Hump with a spirit and enthusiasm that no one expected in this listless, uncaring girl. Just straightening her upper spine brought a desire to exercise other parts of her body. She did the Squat Drill and the Sway and Arch and the Primordial Walk for general development, and her body filled out beautifully. But the first drill was still Joanie's favorite. She considered, she told me quite seriously, that in all my years of research I'd never developed anything quite so useful as the Dowager's Hump.

For her, this was true. She related to this drill more than to others. As one philosopher put it: "It all depends on how you look from where you stand."

WHAT TO DO FOR FALLEN STOMACH

The first thing to be done for a fallen stomach—and also for a sagging colon—is a short fast. I am not an enthusiast for very long fasting, though I have seen remarkable results from fasts lasting 30 days and even longer. For people I attend to, where the responsibility is mine, I approach long fasts with apprehension because a long period without food of any kind can, and sometimes does, demineralize the body. Then there's the very devil to pay, for it's almost impossible to get the patient back to normality after that. I have seen this happen several times. The overlong fast demineralized the patient, the endocrine balance was gone, the erstwhile faster could not get rid of the severe imbalance no matter what was done.

So even while I cannot deny the evidence of my senses, and must admit to witnessing great cures (really *cures,* within the precise meaning of the word) from very long fasting programs, I prefer the conservative approach and advise only short fasts where it appears that the patient needs a physiological rest. In a case of fallen stomach a fast of up to seven days is desirable. In my 40 years' practice, I have never seen anything but good result from a one-week fast.

During the first few days without food, the stomach invariably shrinks. It tends to tighten up. Water, only, is taken during the fast, and this only to quench any thirst that may be present. The human body is not a car radiator; glass after glass of water should not be dumped down its interior. The water, if obtainable, should be distilled. The reason for this is that during the few days of pure physiological rest not even the inorganic minerals in tap water ought to burden the organism.

While fasting, and especially after the fast, the Head-Lift should be done with frequency (in order to lift nerve pressures in the neck). During the day it is recommended that one with a fallen stomach should take 15-minute rest periods in the Knee-Chest position, either in bed or on the floor. This cannot be overdone, thus should be done often, say every two hours. While in the knee-chest position, it is wonderfully helpful to do vigorous Diaphragmatic Breathing in the following manner:

Consciously lift the shoulders so that the ribs are extended, thus opening the chest cage. With your mouth open, pant in the manner of a panting dog. Note the diaphragmatic region of your abdomen as you do this. Just below the breastbone, where the ribs join in an upward curve toward the breastbone, you will see the in-and-out movements of your abdomen. Continue this in-and-out panting motion until quite tired. If you do this properly, the only area of tiredness will be in the diaphragm.

When you break the fast, you have the choice of doing so with small sips of fruit juice the first day or two, or with lightly steamed zucchini squash. If you prefer orange juice, let's say, take about two ounces every two hours the first day and _do not drink it but take it with a teaspoon_, spoon by spoon. In rare instances I have seen patients cramp and do badly even with well-strained orange juice the first day after the fast, but never any untoward reactions with steamed, tender zucchini. After a seven-day fast, one day on fruit juice or squash is enough in most cases, after which one returns to normal food very gradually.

I advise a person with fallen stomach to eat a good-sized raw apple at bedtime for the intestinal bolus it will provide, and because it contains pectin, it is a good intestinal nourisher. For the constipation often associated with this condition, the raw apple helps remarkably. Besides this, I recommend getting the habit of guiding wastes out of the colon by rubbing the outer abdominal walls with open hands. Begin at the right groin and rub upward to the ribs, then across to the flesh just under the left ribs, then downward to the left groin area.

TECHNIQUE FOR PROTRUDING, DROOPING ABDOMEN

This is what people refer to as their "hanging stomach." It is a counter-gravitational condition almost never seen in four-legged animals. It is best handled, and neutralized, by two specific approaches. First, the Diaphragmatic Breathing drill, done in prolonged rather than short periods (because the in-and-out panting movements tend to tighten the abdominal walls), plus—second—the very fine approach to the problem which follows:

Lie flat on your back. Raise your legs with locked knees one after the other. Keep on alternating the legs, each leg extended full length, knees *not* bent. The leverage is greatly beneficial to your abdomen.

While alternating the legs in this manner, each one with locked knee going as high as you can comfortably lift it, place your hand on the flesh of your belly and note what's happening. The rippling interplay of the abdominal muscles is something to observe as they gyrate and squeeze excess fat out of the intercellular spaces. Do this until very tired in the abdominal area, morning and night, but especially at night.

HOW TO STRENGTHEN AN INACTIVE DIAPHRAGM

To repeat a most important item I explained earlier, when as babies we rise from our baby crib to live vertically thereafter, we begin to breathe only with the apex of each lung instead of with the lower lobes *from the diaphragm.* Gravity forces which push down upon us make it quite easy for us, as creatures existing on two feet, to quit using the diaphragm and forget to breathe with it. Thus, this strongest muscle in the male body (and second strongest in the female) becomes almost paralyzed from disuse.

Now we must learn to get it back into full and useful functioning shape. To counter the ill effects of living against gravity this is *an absolute must* if we are to gain and maintain good health. Thus, we must adopt a most important new habit: the habit of breathing with our diaphragm—to strengthen it. And use it to oxygenate our body; aerate us; give us a change-over from stale residual air to clean new air.

Diaphragmatic Breathing is, without a doubt on my part, one of the very best new habits you can adopt. You should do all the things I've researched over the years, and listed in this book, to make up for the bad effects of counter-gravitational living; but if you've convinced yourself that you have time for only one or two drills— which I'll never believe because nobody is too busy to be sick—then the Primordial Walk and this Diaphragmatic Breathing drill are the two essential absolutes. Your wonderful body is ever-willing to supply the wanted miracle tune-up for rejuvenated health, but you must do a few things, especially the following.

Lift your shoulders and do the dog-panting drill with open mouth (as described on page 193). This reoxygenates your body, and oxygen is life. (As mentioned before, breath—not bread—is the staff of life.) With a greater oxygenating capacity, your body can burn up and eliminate accumulated toxic products, clean up your internal plumbing, tune you up for the day's activities.

Now straddle a chair and place your arms on the back of the chair. This both raises your shoulders and permits you to rest your arms at the same time. With both arms thus resting on the chairback which faces you in the chair-straddling position, do the Diaphragmatic Breathing drill with enough vigor that you feel it in the mid-section—the diaphragm.

If you have cold extremities, your cold toes and fingertips will get warm after an energetic drill of Diaphragmatic Breathing. If you suffer from shortness of breath, this is especially *your* kind of activity, one which, fortunately, even the very debilitated person can engage in. Heretofore, you have hardly ever taken a deep breath into your lower lobes with the full aid of the diaphragm. All that residual air in the bottom lobes of your lungs has gone untapped, unused, unchanged. Only when the long distance runner reaches "second wind" does he get through to the full use of his great store of reserve air. Now, standing or sitting and straddling a chair if you are weak or tired, by making this a daily habit you will regularly change the stored air in the lower lungs and be tapping those reserves.

Note: do this drill of Diaphragmatic Breathing while driving your car also. With hands on the wheels raise the tips of your shoulders enough to expand the ribs, then pant vigorously with the mouth open. It will oxygenate you and stir you alive if you feel drowsy. Do not take dangerous drugs to stay awake on long, tiresome trips. Give your diaphragm a workout to revive you and drive the sleepiness out of you.

WHAT TO DO FOR A PROLAPSED UTERUS

In this condition, the female womb has lost its normal position and either dropped or flopped backward or forward. The suspensory ligaments are weak from loss of tone. The effects of living against gravity must be neutralized by some compensatory measures.

There are three ways to reach this desired end, all of them natural and effective. First, the Knee-Chest position several times a day is recommended: 15-minute periods in this position, three or more times daily. Next, frequent and vigorous drills of Diaphragmatic Breathing *while on the knees and chest* help to firm up the abdominal and pelvic viscera. Finally, the somewhat indelicate matter of attempting to suck back the stool. While the woman with a prolapsed uterus is in the Knee-Chest position, and also getting the benefit of Diaphragmatic Breathing while on the knees and chest, she can add the third very helpful element into the program and get the full benefit of everything. To do this, after giving herself a good workout of Diaphragmatic Breathing while in the Knee-Chest position, she follows the energetic breathing drill with that of forcefully drawing back the stool matter—as though she were going to have a bowel movement and must hold it for a time.

This latter move, by the way, also tends to strengthen the vaginal sphincter muscles, a matter of some importance in pleasurable sexual activity, as discussed in chapter 7 under *Sex Specifics.*

In this connection I recall Mrs. B-B, an eminent political lady in her early 50's, whose uterus had dropped to where she could feel it slightly above the vaginal opening with her own finger. By training, she was a woman of great discipline. Very diligently, she followed the three-pronged program given here: 1. Knee-Chest; 2. Diaphragmatic Breathing while on knees and chest during a few 15-minute periods daily; 3. Stool In-Drawing with vigor while on knees and chest following diaphragmatic drills. During the first five days, nothing seemed to happen. Then she merely added the Primordial Walk and the Sway and Arch drill and everything seemed to happen. In only ten days from the start of the program, she felt a recognizable and delightful "pick-up" of the womb. *Pick-up* was exactly the word, in the true etymological sense.

When the lady saw these results, she was sure of her ground and went after the rest of it with a vengeance. To her daily list she added the Dowager's Hump, the Head-Lift and the Squat Drill. Her entire body firmed up. The depressing and enervating "down-weight" of the prolapsed uterus was gone. In the strictest sense, she achieved a miracle body tune-up and rejuvenated health.

HOW TO NORMALIZE AND REJUVENATE YOUR PELVIS

The human pelvis can slip in front. This is a matter that is not generally known. If you have ever jumped from a fence or staircase and landed on your heels with a jolt in the lower spine, your pelvic bowl may have slipped downward in front. It occurs near the junction of the thigh-bone and the pubic bone.

We know that people with sacroiliac and lumbago pains go to

doctors of chiropractic and get relief. But, from time to time, the relief obtained does not last. In a day or two, or a week or two, the sufferer must return with the same problem and nearly the same pain. This state of affairs bothered the fool out of me, and about 15 years ago I started researching the problem.

I asked myself one never-ending question—*why?* Why do these lumbosacral and other low-back problems return when chiropractic doctors are known to be the world's experts in this field? What's being done for these cases that should not be done . . . or what's not being done that should be done? Why is a correction *seemingly* made, and the patient walks out of the doctor's office with reduced or eliminated pain, only to have the same problem return? It cannot be that there are no answers to this. There must be reasons.

There were. The pelvis, I discovered, also slips in front. It happens to every adolescent woman of the Occident. She has developed a front-slipped pelvis merely from going through the up-and-down pelvic strain of changing from high heels to low heels, to high heels to low heels, and so on. Oriental women who wear flat slippers may not have this. This slipping effect, so common in our females from wearing high-heeled shoes, also happens to adult men, and even to young boys, I have found. It's one more price that we pay for living against gravity, and taking our jolts and jars and falls in a counter-gravitational position.

If you have suffered a long-standing low-back problem that has refused to get better and *stay* better, here is the probable reason. When the chiropractic doctor has adjusted your lower back and established structural integrity in your spine, he's surely done a needful and useful work. But, if your pelvis has slipped in front just below the pubic bone, it must also be raised where it slipped. If not, the pull against the spine in back (from the distortion in front) will sooner or later cause the doctor's correction to come undone. For this reason I have evolved—and present here to you—a reasonable and physiologically proper solution to the problem.

THE TECHNIQUE OF LIFTING THE PELVIS

Lie on your back and feel the pubic bone; it's usually right beneath the broad part of the triangle of pubic hair. Feel along the upper rim of this pubic bone until you touch the end of it at the right, and here you press down into the flesh. If your pelvis slipped in front on the right side, here is where you will feel considerable pain when you press the flesh backward toward the spine. Try the end of the pubic bone on the left, on the upper margin of it. Press the flesh here backward into the spine. If the pain you feel is very great on this side (much more than what you felt when pressing down on the right), then this is probably where your pelvis slipped in front.

Now move the side of your hand up along the inner thigh until it's stopped where the thigh joins the pelvis. At this juncture you will find (and feel) a heavy, whipcord-like tendon in *spasm*. This tendon (Gracilis) is sore to the very touch. It needs to be lifted toward the shoulder on that side, which immediately (and phenomenally!) removes the sharp pain that was present at the rim of the pubic bone.

The best way to achieve this lift is to use the edge of one hand up tight against where the thigh joins the pelvis. Let us say that you found the much sharper pain at the right outer rim of the pubic bone, indicating that this is where the pelvis slipped. Slide your right hand up the right thigh to where it joins the pelvis. Let the edge of this hand get up tight into the joining-place. Now your left hand can grasp the wrist of the right lifting hand and aid it in the lifting action. Using both hands in this way, give this underside of the pelvis a boost upward by a straight, steady lift, not by a sharp upward jerk.

Do this several times and rest quietly on the back. Do it most especially at bedtime, thus carrying the value of the lift with you all through the night. By thus correcting the pelvic front slip, you will have nothing more from the front pulling against the backbone and upsetting it. After a week of nightly attention to this technique, you may safely go to the drills that are meant to correct your vertebral problems in the spine. These, as you already know, are the Pelvic Back-Tip, the Sway and Arch, the Dowager's Hump and Squat Drills. It should not be forgotten also that it is always of natural health value to compensate for living against gravity by way of the other drills given in the *Glossary*, chapter 12, plus the oxygenating drills and the programs for purifying the blood chemistry through detoxification.

CHAPTER ELEVEN

How to Apply the Morrison Counter-Gravity Plan and Correct Nervous Tension, Protruding Abdomen, Hernia and Spinal Disc Problems

Are you sick of being sick? That's something I've asked people for years. It was my way of opening the subject, just to explain that they might as well be sick and get used to it until they did one great thing. That one thing is to compensate for the unhealthy effects that gravity has on us.

From nervous tension to flat feet to hemorrhoids, people suffer because of gravity pressures. They are not told to do anything for this; they are told to take pills. Failing this, they undergo what is euphemistically called "surgical repair." This means that what the pills could not mend the surgeon must, in the end, repair. Meanwhile, however, the damage proceeds unhalted because what most people need is not a round-robin of pills but a program that will offset the effects of gravity. That's the *Missing Link* in healing, and that's what they need.

Facing reality, then, all of us suffer from the ill effects of gravity. Counter-gravity diseases and dysfunctions hit us. But what can be done before they hit us? What can we do to stop them from hitting us? Anything? Yes. Very much.

Here in the following pages you can learn what to do. And how to do it.

HOW YOU CAN TREAT NERVOUS TENSION
NATURALLY AT HOME

What is the surest indicator of nervous tension in the human being? Put another way, what is the best indicator of a high-strung nervous system in a person? *It is the anal sphincter.* There are really two sphincters, internal and external, but it'll make it easier if we consider both as one in this kind of book for lay people.

Living the way we do against gravity, the sphincter gets tight. Consider it as a kind of ring of strong rubbery material that can contract and expand. Well, fighting gravity in our upright state as an up-and-down structure, the circular muscle fibers of the sphincter close up tightly as though to *keep the various organs in the body from falling out.*

Thus the key indicator of the tensed human being is the anal sphincter. There's an easy-to-remember rule among those who are truly knowledgeable in matters of the nervous system. The rule is: *The tighter the sphincter, the tenser the man.* In my own work with thousands of patients, naturally paying special attention to their nervous network, I long ago ran into an observation worth noting. Highly nervous and tense patients had anal or rectal openings so very unusually tight that it was difficult even to insert a well-lubricated dilator the size of an enema rectal piece.

HOW TO INFLUENCE THE ORGANS NOT
UNDER CONTROL OF THE WILL

Stretching and dilating the anal sphincter is a most important technique in gaining a *Miracle Tune-Up for Rejuvenated Health.* With this alone you make a giant stride forward to the kind of solid health that comes from having neutralized the force of gravity on the various organs of the body. All you need to do is obtain a rectal dilator and tube of K-Y jelly, or bottle of vitamin E (wheat germ) oil. If you lack a dilator, the ordinary vaginal douche piece will serve very well. The broad end is lubricated and inserted while you are in a knee-chest position or lying on your left side. It is pushed into the rectal opening for a distance of three or four inches; if it goes farther it does no harm, for it can go nowhere to get lost, so do not be alarmed. After insertion, hold it in place for a moment until you feel the sphincter muscles gripping it. After that, the sphincter will hold it as in a vise.

Maintain this position with dilator inserted within the anus for about 15 minutes. Do these 15-minute periods often, particularly at bedtime. People troubled with hemorrhoids and constipation report especially fine results.

I had carefully explained the neurological value of this sphincter-dilating technique to Claude Hammerstone, a high school biology teacher who grasped it completely. He reported the results with high enthusiasm:

"I told my wife to do it because she had crying jags and was nervous," he explained. "That bit about the dilator touching the Impar ganglion of the sympathetic chain and thereby influencing organs not under control of the human will, that was what made my wife itch to try out dilating the anal sphincters. Not only did she cool down, and simmer down, and become a steady, un-nervous person," he added gleefully, "but the dilating program also did wonderful things for her bowels. Quite a change it made from the constipated woman she was."

What the biology teacher failed to add was insomnia. Those who do this technique of dilating the sphincters almost unfailingly report good improvement in dropping off to sleep, and then sleeping soundly. In latter years, I have heartily recommended rectal dilation for insomnia in all age levels.

HOW TO AVOID SITTING POSITIONS
THAT CAUSE BACKACHES

In the pelvic bowl we have the ischia, one ischium on each side, which are our "sitting down bones." They support the weight of the upper body. Formerly, it was an indelicacy to refer to what you sat down upon, and that's probably why the hip bones are still technically called "the innominates"—meaning bones without names.

But they ought to be named, and also emphasized. They are what you must sit on—never on the tailbone (coccyx) or on the lower (lumbar) spine. Why is this so? Because when you sit on the ischia you are sitting straight up on the posterior, without the backbone curving itself into something else. Gravity has the least tiring effect on you when you sit this way. But when you slide off the ischia and slip down onto your spinal end, that's when you tire the most.

So the rule is to sit straight upward. Soft and overstuffed furniture is not recommended; it allows the distorted body to sag instead of acting like a splint-board that supports the body framework. More-over, please note, the size of the chair-seat is of real importance. From front to back it should not be greater than the length of your upper legs from the end of the thighs to the bend of the knees. If you sit for long in a *deep* chair whose seat is far longer than your upper legs, you just must scoot down on your tailbone to rest your feet on the floor. Thus, be sure to sit preferably in a straight-backed chair with a hard, not upholstered, seat. And sit on the ischia only.

WHAT HAPPENS WHEN YOU CROSS
YOUR LEGS OR KNEES

Our habit of crossing the knees is one that stems from standing two-legged against gravity. The four-legged animal never crosses its legs, or needs to. Knee-crossing makes for poor posture. Worse, it tends to tilt the pelvis. Note the person who sits with knees crossed. One hip is tilted higher than the other. To make up for this the lower spinal vertebrae must compensate, and often there occur what are called compensatory scolioses. The misfortune is that one seldom knows that he is doing it; crossing the knees comes so unconsciously. It's a mechanism for easing the strain on the body that comes from existing against gravitational forces. To stop the habit, you must ask members of your family to remind you when they see you doing it.

I once explained to a very brilliant and very corpulent man the demerits of crossing the knees. After hearing the full explanation, he taught me something I needed to know but didn't.

"Why does everyone cross his knees only one way?" he asked. I had not observed this, and said so. "Of course they do," the patient said with conviction. "Just watch them in your waiting room sometime. Always they cross only in one direction. "Oh," he admitted, "they do at times cross the knees the other way, but that's only for a moment's rest. Then, after a very short rest, back they cross to their favorite side."

The man was right. No wonder he was a luminary, a former member of Congress. I began watching for this and found it to be entirely true. And something else, besides. The manner in which people cross their knees can tell us where, or nearly where in their lower spine they have counter-gravity strains and weaknesses. The things one learns from his patients!

HOW TO HELP TIGHTEN VARICOSE VEINS

In all the years since the birth of the healing arts, not very much of value has been researched for what doctors call the varicosities. It is incredible. There are surgical techniques aplenty, one may be sure. And bandages and things to sell you, of course. But hardly anything at all to help the poor varicose vein sufferer *naturally*. This bothered me no end, considering the vast number of people whose veins cannot stand the ceaseless down-pressure of gravity and who are seen walking around with unsightly bulging legs.

Hours of research went into seeking a solution. Despite the great weight of animals like the horse or cow, their legs almost never get varicosed. The answer wasn't hard to find: their weight is distributed equally on a broad base of four legs, while man balances on two narrow feet with all his weight straight up and pounding down on his legs. At last a solution came to hand. When discovered, it was a superbly beneficial one while being also incredibly simple.

Run backward in a pool. Or in a swimming tank or creek. Find a spot where the water is only waist high and run backward with great vigor, raising the knees very high as you run. This is far better than swimming as far as varicose conditions are concerned. As you run backward, with knees raised high, you also get a hydrotherapy massage on the calves of the legs as each leg comes down alternately. If no pool is handy, run backward on the beach or anywhere else. Just be sure there is nothing in back of you to trip you. In the act of running backward, you use muscles not ordinarily employed. These muscles tend to lift the protuberant veins.

If the valves have already broken you cannot, of course, expect them to mend with this drill. In the Bible we are reminded that with God "nothing is impossible," and with this wonderful body of ours the same may be true. I can give you definite reasons why broken veins will *not* be repaired by any backward-running drill; yet there have been patients whose veins had more inner wisdom than I've got. Not knowing my beautiful explanations for why they should not get well, they went ahead and repaired themselves (in rare cases) on running backward. The ancient philosopher was right when he wrote that "the heart knows reasons that reason cannot understand."

Though running backward may not heal varicose ulcers and such far-gone damages, if this program is diligently followed we can almost promise that it will tighten your leg tissues. Even merely lying in a bathtub and working the legs backward with great energy is better than nothing—even this tends to arrest the formation of bulging veins, veins which cannot properly return the blood to the heart, veins which are not performing well against gravity.

HOW TO RECONSTRUCT YOUR FALLEN ARCHES

A person can have low back pains that even the best chiropractic attention does not seem to help. Often this is due to fallen arches which transfer what is called "backwash pain" from the feet to the lower spine. What happens is that when the foot flattens, the keystone bones of the arch drop and pinch a nerve that often runs between them. The pain from this pinched nerve can then go "upstairs" through the branch nerve behind the knee, the next branch through the leg and sciatic notch, finally to the spinal vertebrae themselves.

As soon as the offending bones of the arch are lifted, however, they quit pinching the nerve and consequently no more pain is transferred "upstairs." So what I had to develop was a technique by which the reader, as a lay person, could lift his flat feet all by himself. And I did. What I finally worked out was an effective and simple way (two ways in fact) that anyone can do in his own home.

Stand with your toes turned inward, toward each other, as though you are walking "knock-kneed." In this position do some toe raising—up and down, up and down, up and down. In this "pigeon-toed" position you just can't go up and down energetically without forcing the arches to return to their natural upward-curved position. The seven little tarsals that comprise the arch will naturally work themselves upward, and into place, as you perform this drill.

Now, note this. Do this at bedtime *after* you have performed all other tasks and have no more walking around to do. Take a luke-warm foot bath and do the pigeon-toed drill. Having raised the bones of the arches, you step straight into bed without any walking around or pounding them down during the next few hours. The bones will have been lifted and the nerve pressure freed. Being free of pressure, the nerve can transmit (while you lie horizontally in bed) the functional and healing power to the muscle of the foot that binds the arch together.

The foregoing is the first of the two ways I worked out for this condition, and I can promise you that it accords absolutely with the physiology of the body. Now, for an even more effective way—and again a way that is absolutely consonant with structural physiological needs—try this plan for rebuilding flat feet.

After the tepid foot bath at bedtime, step on an old-fashioned rolling pin. Step on it with both feet (for the sake of balance) even though only one foot needs help. Now roll both feet as far forward and as far backward on the rolling pin as you can. Try to make it from far back at the heels all the way to the toes. This may hurt the arch needing correction, but it's temporary. To keep from falling, hold on to the backs of two chairs, one on each side, as you roll.

Often it takes no longer than 30 days of doing this *with persistence* to rebuild fallen arches. If low back pain bothers you from a "backwash condition," the end of the foot problems means the end of the spinal one also.

WHAT TO DO ABOUT HEMORRHOIDS

Here we deal with congested veins of the rectum. It is doubtful if humans would suffer from this if they did not live against gravity and have to fight it all the livelong day. The operation for "piles" can be serious, and it is never exactly a cure within the natural meaning of the word. One question must be answered: does surgical intervention cure anything? Or does it merely repair an ailment that the doctors, with first chance at it, failed to cure?

Considered from the counter-gravitational standpoint, the outlook for most hemorrhoidal states is hopeful rather than bleak. Glance back to the topic of *Nervous Tension* (page 200) and note what I wrote about rectal dilatation. Use this technique of dilating the anal sphincter for hemorrhoids, and you'll be glad you did. Preferably, settle into the knee-chest position when inserting the dilator. If the hermorrhoids protrude, the well-lubricated rectal piece first guides the veins which hang outside back inside the anal opening. Then the dilator is left in the rectum for 15 minutes or longer.

Additionally, before the rectal dilatation, it is useful to take a Neutral Bath (see *Glossary*). This is the most relaxing and energizing of all bathing techniques if we go by long-lasting effects. Following the rectal dilatation, it is beneficial to apply a plain cold washcloth to the anal area. Most of all, the Primordial Walk, as described in the *Glossary*, should be done with regularity for all hemorrhoidal conditions.

WHAT YOU CAN DO ABOUT A HERNIA

A hernia is a tear or a rupture of tissues, usually muscle tissue. It can occur in many places of the body and in various ways. Often we see cases of umbilical hernia, at the site of the navel. Most hernia cases are those where the floor of the abdomen has torn.

The danger lies in the possibility that a loop of the intestine will protrude through the tear, and then a spasm or contraction of the torn parts may strangulate the protruding part of the gut. Ordinarily, the advice for hernia is an untemporizing, unqualified: *surgical repair.* With this we do not agree for a minute. It is but the advice of those whose training did not include the least notion of natural, counter-gravitational healing. They haven't the foggiest idea of what can be done, and the miracles that can happen, when we rectify the counter-gravitational effects of our mode of living, for their training did not encompass this.

Use of the Slant Board

We advise the use of a common slant-board, with one end of the board raised about 12-14 inches, lying on it with your head at the lower end. If the tear in the belly floor is not a wide, gaping one, nature will endeavor to "sew it together" with its own healing ingredients if we can but bring the severed parts close enough together to make contact. On a slant-board you will reverse gravity. While thus reversing gravity, my advice is that you do the following morning and night, but especially before bedtime.

Raise both legs with knees locked and do a "flutter-kick," which is a stiff-legged up and down motion within a rather short distance span. Your feet should criss-cross each other and move no more than 18 inches, back and forth, back and forth. This forces the region of the groin and floor of the abdomen to work, bringing the muscles more nearly together. Hopefully, the torn, severed edges come very close to each other.

Now, with legs raised the same way (knees not bent), do a scissor-like motion, which means that you criss-cross from side to side instead of back and forth. Do this until you are tired.

You are ready now for the specific self-aid technique I've devised for this condition. Place two pans of water alongside you beside the slant-board, one containing water as hot as can be borne without burning the skin, the other containing ice water. Have a washcloth in each basin of water. First, apply the hot washcloth to the abdominal tissues directly over the hernia. This causes the inner parts to dilate (heat relaxes), and fresh blood nutrition flows into the dilated torn areas. After four minutes of heat, remove the hot cloth and at once whip on the very cold cloth. This contracts the underlying tissue, squeezing the blood out of the parts.

As the parts contract they tend to *come closer together.* If the torn parts come close enough together, the body's natural healing forces begin a self-mending process, like the formation of a scar in a deep cut. Keep applying the cold cloth for half the time of the heat application: two minutes. Repeat several times—hot washcloth 4 min., cold 2 min., hot 4, cold 2, and so on.

Having done this at bedtime, you will be lying for the next few hours with your weight off your feet. To help further, raise the foot of the bed about six inches by placing blocks or a few books under the legs.

This program, even all by itself, may cause you to avoid hernial surgery. But there are other valuable self-aids for you. *Generally*, you should also do the Head-Lift drill and the rest of my strongly advised Miracle Body Tune-Up program for Rejuvenàted Health, for this will strengthen other parts of the body at the same time in a general way. *Specifically*, however, here are other workable ways to avoid surgery.

ROLL YOUR THIGHS OUTWARD AND UP

In the *Glossary*, you will find this listed as the Abduct Thighs drill, but here it is offered for hernia cases specifically. This is a way of "abducting" your own upper leg muscles; and in many hernia cases it has been found to be almost a miracle form of self-aid. By flexing the knees and rolling both of your thighs outward and up—as though trying to roll the flesh of the thighs around the femurs—you tend to relax the torn area and promote healing. I would advise your doing this Abduct Thighs drill just before the alternating hot-cold cloth applications. If you like, do only the one thigh on the side of the hernia, although both sides are beneficial in most cases.

DO NOT SIT MORE THAN 20 MINUTES
IN ONE POSITION

Because we live in defiance of the law of gravity we must do something about compensating for it. One thing I am sure we can do to wipe out the ill effects of gravity on our body is not to sit longer than 20 minutes at a time in any one position. Sitting without moving for a long time fixes us in a counter-gravity position. The force of gravity upon our organs forbids this. The only time when you are allowed to stay put for hours in the same position is when you are in bed—horizontally positioned.

I am not aware that any other author or researcher anywhere has come to this conclusion or advises this. But I can report one thing; namely, that when I decided that it is not structurally healthy for the human body to remain fixed in one position for over 20 minutes, and began counseling patients to do the right thing about it, many of the ill effects of gravity evaporated.

Here is specifically what I advise. Listen to the wisdom of the body and learn to appreciate what has lately been called "body time." With your blood flow and nerve impulses forever having to work in a straight uphill road, against gravity, the way to prevent their getting frozen or "fixed" in turgid anti-gravity hardships is to shake them up every little while. Move about every 20 minutes or so.

I can recommend two ways that work very well. When arising from a chair after sitting a long time, immediately get pelvic action going by doing the One-Spot Walk, which is standing in one spot and alternately raising the heels (see *Glossary*). This gets the sacroiliac joints working, swings the pelvis beneficially and *makes the transition from the sitting-down to the standing-up state.* By all means this should be done first thing on rising out of bed, for the same reason—to make the transition from the horizontal of sleeping to the vertical of your counter-gravity workaday life. Also, whenever you have been seated long and rise with an urge to stretch (overcoming, unconsciously, the turgidity of counter-gravity positions), do this One-Spot Walk instead of, or in addition to, stretching. Even if you are too lazy to do this, you should at least get up from your reading position every 20 minutes, or rise from your chair whenever the TV commercials are on, and give yourself a little change of position—if only walking around your chair before sitting down again.

Walk a Bit During TV Commercials

The other way is to bounce up at TV commercial time and do a little Primordial Walk. This is the best way. It will compensate for counter-gravitational ill effects on the body better than anything I know. When reading or sewing or doing anything in the same position for a long time, do not allow gravitational forces to build turgidity into your vessels. Do not sit for longer than 20 minutes in the same place. Move around and shake yourself up. It is insurance for longer life and fewer counter-gravitational ailments.

THE PRIMORDIAL WALK: NATURE'S COUNTER-GRAVITY TUNE-UP MIRACLE

This program of walking on hands and feet (not merely hands and knees), along with the Diaphragm Breathing drill (see *Glossary*), I consider the most important of all things you can possibly do to gain and maintain health.

If a sick person, who's really sincere about winning back his health, were to ask me what three little simple things I could advise for him (because he had no time to do more), I would advise the following: 1. The Head-Lift, because this tends to de-compress the discs in the neck and lift pressures off nerves. 2. Diaphragm

Breathing, because when this is done vigorously and frequently the body reoxygenates and renews itself. 3. Primordial Walk because this, more than any other one activity, tends to return the body to its original, natural, horizontal and non-gravity-fighting state of health.

The Primordial Walk means walking on all fours; yes, crawling on hands and *feet,* to re-establish postural rightness and structural (mechanical) integrity of the body. Pick out the longest hallway in your house, or the largest room that's free of interfering furniture, and crawl until tired. Crawl as a young animal would.

Needless to say, it should not be done in the presence of others. Being a biped at all other times, you cannot expect to be graceful doing this on all fours. But, curiously, this Primordial Walk tends to build gracefulness into the organism. Its value lies in your having to *use all the muscles and ligaments, tendons, cartilages of the body,* giving them all a workout. If at the same time you also reoxygenate the system with proper Diaphragmatic Breathing and do the other counter-gravity and nerve-pressure-releasing drills in this miracle tune-up program, the primordial activity helps all the more.

Caution: This should not be done by extremely weak or debilitated persons—for them the proper diaphragmatic breathing alone is sufficient *at first.* But as soon as strength returns, and by use of this program it returns with amazing speed in most cases, just a few steps of Primordial Walk may be tried without fear. As the organism responds, more of the walk on hands and feet may be tried. A state of euphoria may be expected to follow even the smallest attempt at primordial walking; "primordial" because it hearkens back to our earliest beginnings as walking creatures. With daily persistence, in but a short time, you may expect to feel exhilarated and benefitted by this activity.

Note: The Primordial Walk should be done *after* the Head-Lift and Diaphragmatic Breathing and all other drills in the program. When done after the other activities, walking on hands and feet tends to work the various parts of the body back into adjustment. However, what may be done following the Primordial Walk is any specific drill for the correction of nerve pressures, such as the Dowager's Hump, Sway and Arch and Pelvic Back-Tip (see *Glossary*).

WHY DO "CHILDREN'S DISEASES" APPEAR WHEN THEY DO?
(How Gravity Causes Children's Diseases)

When is the first time that we begin living against gravity? It's when we begin trying to pick ourselves up in the baby crib, isn't that so? We are horizontal beings until we begin to feel enough strength in our back muscles to try lifting ourselves. At first we cannot make it.

But after a while we try again, and finally we manage to defy gravity by sitting upright.

But, please note, those first few times our back muscles are not yet strong enough for the task of holding us aloft. Maintaining all that weight against gravity is a strain, so things in our backbone tend to buckle. One or more vertebrae shift from their normal position. As they shift, they press upon nerves. When this happens, the organs which are served by such nerves are deprived of their energy and functional power. The organs depend on receiving working energy and directional impulses by way of the nerves, and when the nerves are pinched by shifted vertebrae the impulses cannot get through. Thus—being deprived of what they need because of nerve pressures—the organs get sick.

I have not personally researched what is suggested here. Being occupied with other physiological investigations, this was earmarked for a future time. But other matters intruded themselves and this was never done.

The thought, however, keeps nibbling and gnawing at me insistently. What theory have the healing sciences evolved, other than the above, to explain why the ailments labeled as "Children's Diseases" plague the children *just then.* Why?—unless it's *just then* that the nerve pressures first occur as the result of beginning to live against gravity.

In the healing arts we must have sensible working ideas as to why things happen in our bodies—what *unnatural* things we do, or habits we acquire in defiance of natural laws, that change natural functional *ease* into *dis*-ease. As related to the "children's diseases," what else has happened at that time to make the little ones vulnerable to disease except nerve pressures from defying gravity? It is just after they have learned to sit up, and exist in a counter-gravitational state, that they have acquired for the first time in their lives the strains (and falls and bruises and jars) that constitute the toll exacted for living against gravity—that's when the "febrile diseases" attack them. If there is any better working theory in this area from any healing-arts source, I'd be mighty pleased to hear it.

HOW TO KEEP FROM GETTING SHORTER
WITH ADVANCING AGE

You have already read earlier in this book, in a discussion of this subject, that human beings tend to get shorter in stature with advancing age. This is because the flexible cartilages (discs) between the vertebrae thin down with the years. Bearing all that bodily weight above them, and ceaselessly bearing down and even pounding down upon them, flattens them. Therefore, it would be a great, health-inducing thing to stretch out the spine in order to make more room for these discs between the vertebrae. Doing this would act to decompress the discs.

Is there a way whereby we can overcome this disc compression? The best way I've ever found is hanging by the arms from loops into which you can slide your wrists. Just to hang dead weight and stretch, stretch, s-t-r-e-t-c-h along the spine, very markedly tends to widen the intervertebral spaces where the discs are. If there is one place where gravity-living takes its daily toll, it's right there—all that weight upon the discs between the vertebrae, because we live straight up-and-down rather than on four legs. (You can see at once that these discs would not be compressed by any great weight-bearing chores if your body were horizontal.) And if there is one way to reverse all that down-pressure on the discs, it is by hanging from loops strung around the wrists.

Find some old, unused belts and loop them around a pipe or chinning bar in the doorway. Slide your wrists into the loops and let go. Allow the entire body weight to let go and just hang, hang, hang without effort. You will feel the pull or stretch at first in your arms and elbows. Then the wonderful feeling of being stretched will transfer to the spine and you will almost be able to tick off each vertebra as it tractions, comes loose and somewhat separated. While this happens, you will be overcoming the effects of gravity; making room for the transmission of impulses and fluids through the spinal nerves and vertebral blood vessels; conceivably even making you somewhat taller.

This is a highly recommended technique by which you can begin to overcome the strains and stresses accumulated by your body throughout the years of living against gravity. By thus returning your body to a state of structural and mechanical rightness you are, in the words of Dr. J.E. Goldthwait in *"Essentials of Body Mechanics in Health and Disease,"* making "correct function of your organs possible [because you are] giving the organs a chance to do the job for which they are intended."

THE BEST TECHNIQUES FOR OVERCOMING GRAVITY AILMENTS

Remember to remember the following.

The Head-Lift drill, because it offers the best way in the world that I know to take pressures off nerves of the neck. These are the nerves which nourish the tissues of the face and head, and direct their function also. Out of our five special senses, no fewer than four depend upon freely operating cranial nerves. Although these do not themselves traverse the neck in the manner of other spinal nerves, they are very greatly influenced toward health when nerve pressures are lifted in the neck. So, for facial and head problems, do the Head-Lift.

The Dowager's Hump drill for round shoulders and a forward-stooping upper spine, which stooping condition is one great effect of existing in defiance of gravity. With this drill, you can free impingements in the nerves of the upper spine and prevent a "hump" from forming. Just touch both palms in back of you and turn the elbows inward as hard as you can.

The Knee-Chest position in which you rest face down, with kneecaps and chest upon the floor or bed, to reverse the down-strain of gravity upon your stomach and other vicera. For increased value you should merge this position with some workout of the diaphragm, as in the drill that follows.

The Diaphragmatic Breathing drill (for the inactive diaphragm) which is one of the most important techniques in the Miracle Body Tune-Up for Rejuvenated Health. This is so because, when you raise your arms and pant through open lips (like a dog's panting), you reoxygenate the entire system and give yourself renewed life. Although there are some drills which can conceivably be overdone (such as the Squat Drill), this one may be done as often as you like—and with benefit.

The Nervous Tension Technique which is that of Dilating Anal Sphincters. This is done with a plain vaginal douche piece that is well lubricated with oil or Vaseline Petroleum Jelly or K-Y jelly and inserted for about 15 minutes, while you lie on the left side or in the knee-chest position. If available, the commercial rectal dilators serve even better. Young's Rectal Dilators come in graduated sizes, beginning with the small one for infants and going on to the largest size the rectal opening can accommodate.

The Varicose Veins treatment of Running Backward in a Pool, raising the knees high while doing so.

The Fallen Arches method of using a plain Rolling Pin (or two cylindrical bottles placed end to end) to lift the collapsed arch-bones. This is done right after a tepid foot bath just before bedtime. It is always advisable for low back pains that persist despite treatment.

The Primordial Walk is that of walking, or crawling, on hands and *feet* (not knees) to overcome the ill effects of counter-gravitational living. This, along with frequent and vigorous Diaphragmatic Breathing, plus lifting the head off the neck and shoulders by means of the Head-Lift, can very nearly, without anything else, return much of anyone's lost health.

And, lest you forget, "remember to remember" not to cross your knees (because that tilts the pelvis) as an unconscious shifting of weight to rest from the constant *uprightness* of living against gravity; and remember also to do the One-Spot Walk and Squat Drill and Pelvic Back-Tip and Sway and Arch from time to time. All of them are incalculably valuable techniques for overcoming the ailments caused by gravity.

BENEFITS OF COUNTERING EFFECTS OF GRAVITY

Here ends a very important chapter indeed. In learning about the toll that we pay every day merely because we live against gravity, we enter a new dimension in the science of healing. We learn something that the world must positively know: how to overcome the health-destroying effects of counter-gravity existence.

It can be done. But we must know how to do it. We must *learn* how. And until we learn, as set forth here, and until we abandon the chimera of being able to correct the body's mechanical faults by taking chemical ingredients or products (drugs, injections, and so forth), we will continue being sick. It is too easy in our society to become bedazzled by the magical things that the chemical interests wish to sell us—the TV and radio announcers have such beautifully-trained, ingratiating voices and come at us with such mellifluous language rhythms that it's hard to resist them. But they are not doctors, they're salesmen, and resist their blandishments we must.

For our ills that are caused by mechanical factors such as living against gravity and sustaining nerve pressures, we need mechanical aids rather than the chemical ones that the pharmaceutical interests wish to sell us. Until we learn this completely, and act accordingly with intelligence, we are doomed. Doomed to being forever sick and forever needing more hospitals, and ever-more hospitals, out of all proportion to our rising population, in order to care for the ever-increasing load of sick people.

Here we have been listening to the wisdom of the body, and doing something about it. Ben Franklin used to say that "nature cures and the doctor pockets the fee," and here we have been learning how to help ourselves (help the body cure itself) *naturally*. To be able to cure itself, the machine must be in proper mechanical working order;

there is no other way by which the organs have the chance to do the work for which they are intended. This is a prime lesson of the body. If you ask yourself again, "Am I sick of being sick?" the answer is that you will be, or remain, sick until you go at the body's ills mechanically, not chemically.

YOUR BODY IS FIRST A MACHINE,
THEN A CHEMICAL FACTORY

Your body produces its required chemicals, as insulin or adrenalin, if it is in mechanical order. If there is a mechanical nerve pressure on a nerve to the stomach's peptic glands, this *mechanical* factor prevents the production of a *chemical* and you have dyspepsia. If the force of gravity interferes *mechanically* with the workings of the pancreas, this mechanical factor halts the production of insulin and you have diabetes, truly a *chemical* deficiency. If the straight up-and-down weight of your body bears abnormally on the supra-renal capsules, this *mechanical* factor may disturb the manufacture of adrenalin and give you hypo-adrenia—a disease of a *chemical* nature. This points to one lesson within the wisdom of the body: that we must attend to the body's mechanical ills first. Yet everywhere the hospitals and treatment centers are geared to treating the chemical factors with drugs and sera and vaccines and injectibles—so is it any wonder we are sick and that degenerative sicknesses are rising?

The lessons are simple. The body is a machine. It is a machine that manufactures drugs and ingredients for the operation of its various parts. Like any machine, it has moving parts and a functional center of gravity. In common with other such machines, it can be jolted or jarred out of mechanical adjustment; after which, of course, it loses its maximum functioning ability. Even a stationary machine with just a few moving parts in it (an electric fan, refrigerator, or toaster—which remains stationary where you place it) gets out of mechanical order occasionally. But the human body has many moving parts (over 200 bones, three times that many muscles, ligaments, tendons, cartilages), and heaves and falls and strains and jars and jolts itself instead of being stationary, so it gets out of mechanical order more often. When the human body is for any reason yanked out of mechanical whack, it cannot perform its chemical jobs of elaborating and manufacturing the needed ingredients for health, growth and self-repair.

WHY PEOPLE REMAIN SICK

Now, it is easy to understand why our sick friends have been treated for 20 years and are still sick. They had mechanical ailments and went for such ailments to a chemical (drug-dispensing) doctor. If you go to the dentist, you cannot be fitted for glasses; if you visit the pyschiatrist, you will not have your teeth pulled; if yours is the wrong doctor, you cannot expect to get the right treatments. Most human ills are *originally* triggered by mechanical factors, of that I haven't the faintest doubt (since we live against gravity).

With such ailments of original mechanical causation, our sick friends have gone for 20 years to doctors trained in treating chemical imbalances. Naturally, then, they are still sick. How can any doctor mend them with chemicals when they need mechanical corrections? At best, he can only divert the symptoms, and make it seem as if a change was being made, but it must be a temporary, and sometimes harmful, change if the original cause is not treated. In seeking a doctor, we must learn to distinguish between two kinds: doctors of *causes,* and doctors of *effects.*

EVEN THE BEST FOOD MAY NOT BE HELPFUL FOOD

A final note which the reader may find astounding, or even exasperating. The entire truth is that *the potential value of any food is not its actual value.* It must first be appropriated and utilized; then a food is translated into good bone and muscle and nerve and gland tissue. But if one's gravity ills interfere with the nerve power to the digestive organs, for example, even the best foods cannot be utilized. This explains why so many of our friends who buy only the best foods and eat just exactly "according to Hoyle" are still sick. It explains also why I am giving all this attention to, and concentration upon, the Miracle Tune-Up to overcome the ill effects of counter-gravitational living.

Now, note well, there's a reverse side to this. Great and sane and wise as it is to eat good food and live in a salutary environment, the unbelievable truth is that when the body is in proper *mechanical* condition, and the gravity tolls are compensated for, a very high state of health is possible even without the best foods or the best environment. The body can "make do" with poor foods and a bad atmosphere, almost beyond imagination, if the gravity forces are reversed and there are no nerve-line pressures blocking the flow of Life Force to the various organs.

THE MAN WHO WOULDN'T EAT ANY "RABBIT FOOD"

In this connection, Robert Wybie, fictitiously named, was a spoiled-brat adult, accustomed to having his own way and a disagreeable patient from the start. "I won't be dieted or fiddled with," he said straightaway. "Just do your folderol on my body and let me go. If you want me to do anything on my own, you've got the wrong boy."

Ordinarily, I'd have shown this fresh one the door in preciously short order. But his family had been longtime patients and very good ones. They begged that I humor the undisciplined, brassy fellow, which I did. And he got well!

Of course, he may have cheated by eating on the sly some foods he told me he'd never touch. "No rabbit food for me!" he insisted with unruly emphasis, and I think he meant it. However that was, I know what I have seen so many times in other cases. The nerve impulses which newly reached his organs after years of pressures on the nerve pathways, that's what accomplished the cure. With a kind of magic inherent in the body, the nerve impulses managed to convert the steaks and potatoes and apple pie and coffee he ate into good muscle tissue and blood tissue and all the rest. I have learned long ago this lesson I wish to share with you. *Never underestimate the Health Power flowing to organs by way of nerve pathways when the body is mechanically correct, free of nerve pressures and faulty mechanical relationships.*

Obviously, the body can do far better with appropriate foods: organically grown fruits and vegetables, non-hydrogenated fats, assimilable proteins (not more than 50 grams daily as explained elsewhere), and good unpolluted air to breathe and so forth. We make no brief for sad souls who insist on consuming only the demineralized and denatured foodstuffs that their jaded appetites crave, for in time their bodies must suffer.

We are, in fact, what we eat. The human organism cannot build without building materials of a usable kind. But when the body is ailing, and the right foods are not taken or available, even bad foods can be converted to good uses. The functional energy which reaches the organs by way of the nerves can, at least temporarily, make use of whatever is available.

So long as nerve power flows to the digestive apparatus without interference, the body can somehow "make do" with supplies at hand, even while hungering for better materials. Just as a calcium-poor pregnant woman will somehow provide the developing fetus with the needed minerals, even if they must be taken out of her own teeth, so will the human body utilize even poor foods for a good purpose *if* the power to accomplish this reaches the organs through free, un-pinched nerves.

We trust that the reader will never forget what he read here. Without a mechanically correct body there can be no health. And without health there can be no other deep satisfaction in life.

CHAPTER TWELVE

Glossary of Missing Link
Techniques and Programs

For your convenient reference in tuning up your body for rejuvenated health, this dictionary of "Missing Link" factors embraces the following:

A — How to make up for the harmful effects of living against gravity.

B — How to set the body right mechanically.

C — How to set the body right chemically.

D — How to improve the oxygenating capacity of the body.

E — How to eliminate nervous tension.

A: *Techniques and drills by means of which you can make up for the harmful, down-pulling gravity strains on the body.*

1. Primordial Walk. This is perhaps the most important single piece of research I have ever developed. Along with the drill for diaphragmatic breathing (see under "D"), it is the most "missing" and most beneficial of get-well doctoring techniques. What it consists of is merely walking on hands and feet. Not hands and knees, but hands and *feet.* It compensates for much of our counter-gravitational strains and stresses and provides strengthening activity to just about *all* the muscles, ligaments, tendons and cartilages of

the body. Pick out the largest room or hallway in your home and walk on all fours, the kind of walking done primordially, by your first ancestors. If weak or old or greatly debilitated, do a very small bit of this Primordial Walk at first. It soon strengthens one so that he desires to do more. Or confine yourself to diaphragmatic breathing until you feel somewhat stronger, then try the Primordial Walk.

2. Knee-Chest Position. This should be the favored rest position at all times. The chest or breastbone rests on the bed or floor while the lower spine and tailbone are supported by the knees. This causes the body to slant from head upward to loins, which is counter to gravity. Women with fallen wombs find comfort and benefit from this. Men and women with prolapsed stomachs are helped by the knee-chest position. The diaphragm in all of us benefits greatly.

3. Head-Down Position. This consists of lying crosswise on the bed with the head hanging over the edge of the bed. It is best to have the chest on the bed up to the collarbones, then the neck and head extend downward over the bed. The mere weight of the head provides a good neck stretch as it hangs loosely downward. The important nerves and blood vessels that traverse the neck to reach the body are thus given the benefit of counter-gravitational ease. One may spend as much time as desired in this position. If time passes too slowly, with nothing to do while thus hanging the head, it is possible to read a large-print book in this position, the book resting on the floor below you.

4. Spinal Disc Decompression . . . . Hanging suspended from loops. As we grow older, we are usually shorter than in our youth because the discs which separate the spinal vertebrae tend to get thinner with the weight and pounding-down of the body above. The force of gravity compresses the spinal discs. Hanging suspended from a couple of wrist-loops does more to decompress the discs than anything else ever invented by man. Just attach a chinning bar in your doorway, or even the limb of a tree will do. Throw two loops over the bar and fix your wrists firmly into them. Now merely hang loosely, without straining, just dead weight. Imagine that you are a

washed-out rag doll. You will feel the down-pull first in your elbows, then in the arms. Finally the decompressing effects are felt in your spine itself. The discs are spreading apart. You cannot overdo this. It will help you gain and maintain health.

5. Abduct Upper Thighs. This further assures the correct repositioning of the entire bowl of the pelvis under the spinal column, thus serving as a good supporting platform for the body above. Just lie on your back with knees drawn up, feet flat on the bed or floor. Reach your hands down to the inner side of each thigh, high up near the crotch. Now merely roll the flesh of the thigh around the thigh-bone, *outward* and somewhat *upward*. Don't try to rotate the bone, only the flesh of the thigh around the bone. Do it lightly. Do this at night just before retiring.

6. Run Backward in Pool. The blood in the veins of our legs has a straight uphill climb to get back to the heart. The pressure of gravity is severely against the circulation here, and we get bulging varicose veins. The very best way to get at this condition *naturally* (avoiding surgery and injection techniques) is to run backward in a pool. Lift the knees high as you do this and feel the water massage the calves, treating yourself to a hydrotherapy workout at the same time. Run backward rapidly for best results. Barring a pool, run backward on the beach or anywhere. This puts into play the structures of the leg that need help. In addition to this technique for the natural counter-action to harmful gravitational pulls on your body, try stretching the Achilles' tendons back of the ankles. Just lie in bed or on the floor with the feet elevated a little on a pillow or a few books. Lying thus on your back, curl the toes upward toward your shins. Feel the stretch in the strong wiry tendons coming up the back of your legs from the heels. Do this rapidly and frequently. Do it especially at bedtime.

This counter-gravitational portion of the *Missing Link in Healing* is unknown and ignored in all doctoring professions presently holding forth. Until we compensate every day for the harmfulness of counter-gravitational living, however, we cannot reasonably expect any significant downturn in presently rising heart disease, cancer, mental illness, diabetes, arthritis, epilepsy, muscular dystrophy, multiple sclerosis, cystic fibrosis, cerebral palsy, renal degenerations, or even the common cold.

B: *Techniques and programs by means of which you can help the body get into a state of mechanical rightness, aiding pinched nerves.*

1. Head-Lift. To lift mechanical pressures on nerves and other structures of the neck the best home method is to raise the head "off the neck and shoulders." Do this sitting or standing. Place open palms and extended fingers in contact with your lower jaws, the fingers extending backward to just under the mastoids. Now merely lift straight upward, and turn the head as you lift. Turn to your full limit of motion, not forgetting to lift meanwhile, and then give the head and neck a little extra stretch as you keep lifting. Do this in both directions, turning *and lifting* the head off the neck as far as you can. This cannot be overdone. If you are too weak to do this, another person may help at first. Nighttime is the best time for this; what you gain at bedtime you will take to bed with you, to benefit you through the night. In a short time, you will notice that you can turn the head farther in each direction, and with markedly less strain, as you release nerve pressures by this Head-Lift.

2. The Neck Traction. Lie on your back and have someone, standing behind you, grasp the jaws and back of the head in cupped hands and pull backward in a straight line. The head is pulled toward the person who is helping you, pulled as though to separate the head from the shoulders. This need be done only two or three times. The traction is intermittent: pull and release, pull and release, and so on. After the tractioning, the helper allows you to remain resting on your back. This enables the newly-separated structures to get accustomed to the position where they no longer press upon nerves.

3. Dowager's Hump. Clasp both hands together behind you with palms touching. Lace the fingers of both hands if you like. Now roll your elbows inward as vigorously as you can. Try touching the elbows if possible. Note how this unslouches the shoulders, thrusts the chest forward,

gives the pectoral muscles a workout. The Dowager's Hump tends to release nerve pressures in the upper spine in the same way that the Head-Lift and Neck Traction did this for nerve pressures of the neck. This may be done often, especially at night.

4. Sway and Arch. To give yourself "an adjustment" and aid in un-pinching nerves in the upper and middle spinal column, get on your hands and knees, supported thus at four points. Now try to achieve as deep a swayback as you can, hollowing out a concavity in your backbone. Then arch upward as high as you can. Continue until tired. (When thoroughly tired, I recommend that you lower yourself to the Knee-Chest position for a rest period.)

5. Pelvic Back-Tip. To lift pressure off the nerves of the lower back and off protruding spinal discs, lie on the back and flex knees toward the chest and shoulders. First, with open cupped hand on the left knee, press the knee as far as you can toward the left shoulder. Then do the same with the other knee. Finally, with one hand on each knee, press both toward the tips of the shoulders. Press down hard, but do not jerk—not ever. This may be done on the floor or on a hard, resistant bed. It tends to replace the pelvis in the mechanically correct position under the spinal column, not tipped forward at the hip-bones as it is in almost everyone. So long as we live against gravity, we tend toward getting mechanically malpositioned; so this drill ought to be done all one's lifetime.

6. One-Spot Walk. This is a necessary *transitional* technique, one that makes the proper mechanical change from the horizontal position of sleep to that of sitting or standing. Feet are about four inches apart, parallel with each other. Now you raise the heels alternately while the other foot is flat on the floor. Try not to jar the heel as it goes down; better to *almost* touch the floor going down with the heel, but start up again before you do. This drill is like walking in one spot; the foot movements are the same, but you do not travel. Place your hands on hips as you do this One-Spot Walk and note how the lower spine articulates. You are acclimatizing the sacroiliac joints and lower spine to the upright (against gravity) position, and should do this unfailingly upon rising in the morning, or from a daytime nap.

7. Squat Drill. Because of mechanical imperfections, the average human spine is weak and hurting and inadequate. This Squat Drill will strengthen the lower backbone, and make it adequate, better than anything ever invented. Stand with feet about 14 inches apart, heels touching the floor. Now do some knee bending, but this time it's more of a squat because you do not raise the heels off the floor. Squat down as far as you can go (as though for a bowel evacuation in the forest). Hold hands out to the side as you rise (for balance) and try to raise your body without leaning the trunk forward. This means you do not lift your weight with the knees or leg muscles but with the muscles of the lower back. Come up from the squat position kind of backwards—as though falling backward. Do it close to a wall, so if you do lose balance and fall, the wall will stop you from getting hurt. This can be overdone; it is a powerful drill. So start with a mere three squat-and-lift movements morning and night. Increase one on each succeeding week. In six months you should be doing 20, where you should hold it. By this time your lower back muscles will be strong enough to meet every challenge.

Setting the body mechanically right is the province of the chiropractic profession, whose doctors should be consulted when professional help is required. Formerly, osteopaths also dealt with the body's mechanically-caused ailments, although in a relatively imprecise way because they were trained to move almost every articulation that could be made to snap and crackle instead of pinpointing the exact nerve pathways that needed nerve-pressure release. Nowadays, most osteopaths hold forth as "physicians and surgeons" and confine themselves to the drugging techniques used by their allopathic counterparts. (A medical writer in a recent book wrote that anyone labeling himself as both a physician and surgeon was immediately suspect, for it takes a whole lifetime to be either one or the other.) Years ago, when needing chemistry imbalances dealt with, one went to an allopathic medical man, and when needing his body adjusted back into mechanical balance he went to either a doctor of chiropractic or osteopathy. Now he does not have that choice. For tampering with the body's chemistry, it's a medical person or an osteopath; and for mechanical nerve-pressure correction, it has to be a doctor of chiropractic—for no other doctor is trained to do the latter.

C: *Techniques and drills with which to get the body chemically balanced, detoxify the system and purify the blood.*

1. The Fasting Physiological Rest. Since all of us seem to eat wrongly at times, the body becomes a storehouse of accumulated, uneliminated poisons. The best way to detoxify the body and at the same time purify the bloodstream is to fast for a given period. I recommend a period of three days to a week or ten days, which is a short fast, really. I have at times directed much longer fasts but prefer the shorter one as safer, despite the fact that I have seen almost incredible results from very long fasts and cannot deny the evidence of my senses; but at times a long period of abstinence from food demineralizes the system and this is a serious consequence devoutly to be avoided. Moreover, if the one-week fast does not do all that is required, one may eat for a week after the fast and return' to another for a second week—a program that I myself follow in my occasional fasts. The fast, however, must be a perfect *physiological rest.* This means going to bed and staying there except for bathroom requirements. No reading the books you've missed (eye strain uses energy needed for rebuilding the damaged tissues during a fast); no radio going, for noise can be a pollutant and enervates the body also. No writing letters, talking to visitors, and so forth. Just taking a week off to do *nothing.* No drinking either except a little water when there is thirst. Thus, with full physiological rest, the organism's energy is used entirely for healing purposes.

2. The Monodiet. This is the method of eating only one food at a meal. As much as one desires, but only of that one food. If you eat tomatoes, that's it for the meal. If it's grapefruit for breakfast, have five if you like, but nothing else. Doing this for a week or two, further rests the digestive organs following a short fast.
The best combination of foods is no combination at all; thus, those formerly troubled by combining foods wrongly give the body a chance to straighten out. During a week, one may have as many as 21 different foods, so

this isn't the severe program it may seem. I advise only fruits for breakfast: for seven days the choice may be from among these, taken alone each day—oranges, grapefruits, grapes, watermelon, cantaloupe, apples, pears, cherries, persimmons, papaya, honeydew. For lunch I usually recommend a small starch meal during this mono-diet period: bananas (only) or fresh corn, potato (with cold-pressed corn oil added), barley soup, whole rice, yams, coconut, parsnips, carrots, whole grain bread. In the evening, the protein (just two ounces of one kind only) may be taken with a salad of green, leafy vegetables either whole or blended in a liquefier. Choose from among almonds (whole or ground), avocado, sunflower seeds, wheat germ, cottage cheese, pecans, walnuts, soy sprouts, eggs (only two per week).

Observing this monodiet for a week or two following a proper physiological rest, in my studied view is the most perfect way known to man of cleansing the body and up-grading the blood stream. If coupled with compensating for counter-gravitational living by way of the techniques herein given, and clearing the nerve pathways of pressures, everything in your body that can still recover will recover—as I've observed it and know it.

3. The Inviolable "No" List. No shots taken into your muscles, veins or anywhere else—unless under dire emergency conditions, such as a half-severed leg in an accident (where a morphine injection is warrantable even if you may need to fight off morphinomania later, for the pain itself may kill you). Of what use would cleansing the bloodstream be if again polluted with vile injectibles? Plus the grave danger of anaphylaxis (serum poisoning) from the bloodstream's having to play host to a foreign protein; and also the danger of iatrogenic (physician-caused) disease.

The Salk polio vaccine alone, which has been much praised although diverting polio symptoms to increased heart and kidney disease (in my observation), is composed of ingredients the public would never want injected into human bloodstreams. They are, first, the blood taken from a *diseased* Rhesus monkey, then mixed with 60-odd chemicals foreign to the body, then all of this "refined" by interlarding with a form of formaldehyde. It would serve but small purpose to detoxify with a fast and monodiet, and then take a "shot" of all this into your blood.

Another "No" that should not be violated is the over-eating of mucus-forming foods. Other "No's" are: No high protein meals, no raw eggs (because they tend to coat the intestinal lining); no extremely cold or hot foods; no alcohol.

This area of healing is dealt with by the conventional allopathic medical profession, but very poorly dealt with in my judgment, because it is done with drugs which are synthetic for the most part. These I deem an assault on the human body. They leave an array of other diseases (side effects) in their wake. And they do not even have the virtue of really balancing the body chemistry, detoxifying the system, or purifying the blood for all that. My observation over four decades has been that they, contrariwise, pollute the human bloodstream with foreign protein disease material and weaken human resistance against disease—making disease pyramid.

This area of healing is also dealt with quite naturally and satisfactorily by the doctors in the natural hygiene profession; and somewhat less all-embracingly or satisfactorily, I think, by doctors of the naturopathic profession, both of which professions employ no drugs of any kind. I am convinced, however, that my method, herein given, is the best ever evolved for cleansing the body and upgrading the purity of the bloodstream.

A short fast (or a series of them) with perfect physiological rest, then a monodiet week or two, followed by subsistence on a diet of at least 50 percent unfired food; *this* is man's best answer to a chemically disease-free body. It is noteworthy that the dominant allopathic profession ignores all the other Missing Link factors in healing. But surveys have revealed that American pharmaceutical firms spend between $3,000 and $4,000 *per year per drug-prescribing doctor,* just to keep the drug dispensers enthusiastic about the drug-route method of healing—so what chance do non-drugging professions have with nothing to sell but their services?

D: *Techniques that show how to improve the body's oxygenation.*

1. Diaphragmatic Breathing. This simple drill is only next in importance to the vastly beneficial Primordial Walk with which you counteract the ill effects of gravity on your organs. Here, you merely lift your arms high enough to open the chest cage (separate the ribs) and pant like a dog. Keep the lips apart and pant. Move the midriff as you pant. This is the diaphragm that is given a workout. See it move just where the front ribs come together in front to join under the breastbone. As the diaphragm moves, it is getting stronger. With a strong diaphragm, you draw fuller breaths. Oxygen is life. You tap your lung reserves: that huge reservoir of air that goes mostly unused is being used, finally. Customarily, only the runner who gets his "second wind" reaches this great storehouse of air—now you can do it as a regular thing. With a powerful diaphragm, you will speak and sing better and, best of all, reoxygenate the system every few minutes. With a better oxygenating capacity you burn up toxic products and have less chance of disease piling up in your body.

2. Double-Count Exhalations. This is a beautifully easy way to strengthen the muscles of breathing. It is known that the best method of improving your breathing apparatus is to exhale *under control.* So we have refined it down to this: just count as you inhale, and then count twice as much as you let out the breath. This forces you to exhale under control. If you need a count of six to breathe in and take 12 to let the breath out, then toward the last of the 12 your breathing muscles tighten, they get a workout, they get strong. Do this while walking along, or anywhere.

3. Vitamin E Value. In a polluted world, it is a matter of safety to consume a good natural brand of vitamin E (from wheat germ oil) every day. Besides the beneficial effects listed elsewhere in this book (for the heart, etc.), this vitamin enables you to "make do" with less oxygen. It tends to balance the oxygenating functions. Generally one should take about 200 International Units (I.U.s)

daily. With cardiac problems, twice or three times this amount is not unusual.

4. Bicycle Aloft Drill. This excellent and simple effort for the ailing heart is also an exciter of good breathing. Lie on your back, raise your legs and ride a bicycle upside-down by kicking (winding) your heels. Learn how to take your pulse and do this fast enough to speed up your pulse-rate to around 110. Meanwhile, try to remember to breathe with the diaphragm.

5. Avoid Anti-Perspirants. The human skin is a natural breather. It was made to perspire. I think it is a shameful commentary on those who pose as "Guardians of the Public Health" that they do not prosecute the manufacturers of anti-perspirants. Deodorants are bad enough. But actually to sell something to stop a bodily area from perspiring—that's criminal in my view. Most especially when that area is the underarm breathing-and-exit-valve of the body! For your own deodorizing, if needed, try natural chlorophyll. Buy a few chlorophyll tablets, which are merely compressed alfalfa, flaxseed and such green-stuff. Place in a jar and the water turns green. Use this for a mouthwash or under-arm deodorizer.

This oxygenating portion of the *Missing Link* in *Healing* is not in any serious way dealt with by any of the major healing professions. Physical culturists, however, do deal with oxygenation, but only as a kind of by-product of energetic exercising. Since breath, and not bread, is the staff of life, the imprecise approach to improving the human oxygenating capacity (through exercise) is not in my view sufficient. Better oxygen intake means the burning up of body wastes and direct aid for sub-oxidation conditions. Thus, it should not be a mere side-benefit, as from exercising, but one sought in a direct, scientific approach.

E: *Simple techniques which show how to reduce and eliminate nervous tension.*

1. The Neutral Bath. This technique is simplicity itself, and at the same time unbelievably effective. It works so very well because it is a way by which your entire organism— the framework and musculature and organs and the "you

of you"—can hang suspended between exactly equivalent temperatures. You accomplish this merely by fixing a bath at 99 degrees Fahrenheit. Your body is normally just about the same temperature (98.6). Thus, when you let yourself down as far as the neck into such a tubful of water, the immersed body is suspended between equivalent temperatures. When the temperature around you and inside you is the same, then everything in you that can let go does let go. Your tensions disappear. They evaporate. Your 15 minutes in this kind of Neutral Bath is as restful as half a night's good sleep under other conditions. Just hang a thermometer over the side of your tub and do this. The water will magnify the numbers and you'll be able to control it at 99 degrees. Do this whenever especially tired or nerve-jagged or tense.

2. Dilating the Rectum. Inside the rectum there are two rings of circular muscle fibers called sphincters. Due to their position and function and hook-up with the rest of the body, these sphincters, I have found, reflect the presence or absence of nervous tension in the human being. In seminar classroom sessions with chiropractors all over the nation (in 35 cities of the U.S. plus some in Canada and Europe), I have, in fact, taught it this way: *The tighter the sphincters the tenser the person.* Living against gravity as we do, these muscular rings tighten severely in the highly nerve-tensed person, as though to prevent the organs above from dropping out of the anus.

Thus, dilating the sphincters is an almost magical way of easing nervous tension: and also a way of reaching the organs not under control of the will by way of the autonomic nervous system having sphincter hookups. You can rest in the Knee-Chest position or lie on your left side with the knees drawn up, and insert a rectal dilator into the anus. Lubricate it well with K-Y jelly or white Vaseline Petroleum Jelly or wheat germ oil and just let it glide inward for 3 or 4 inches. It cannot get lost or go anywhere to do harm, so insert the rectal piece with assurance.

If you cannot purchase a Rectal Dilator (sold so-named), use a vaginal douche piece. Let it remain within the rectum for about 15 minutes. If you should happen to fall asleep with the dilator inside, nothing bad can happen; it will be that much more helpful.

I can recommend a brand known as Young's Rectal Dilators, sold in a set of several sizes. Begin with the smallest size, and when it can be inserted with ease, work up to the largest which your anal opening can comfortably accommodate. When withdrawing the dilator, it is useful to insert and withdraw from the external sphincter several times, just going in and out a few times to stimulate sphincter expansion.

This area of the *Missing Link in Healing* is dealt with by hydrotherapists, but not very exactly or scientifically. Dilating the anal sphincters is really a neurological technique, with a rather complicated neurological explanation behind it, that belongs rightfully in the chiropractic profession, although not employed as often as it deserves.

It is useful to understand one thing regarding the *Missing Link* approaches and techniques in the field of helping the sick get well. That one thing to know is this: *Dealing with only a single portion of the Missing Link 5-part (A-to-E) program given above is not enough to get people to gain and maintain health.* All of the above constitute the *Missing Link in Healing,* and all are desperately needed in our world of rising degenerative diseases.

If I were to choose one portion of the *Missing Link* ahead of the others it would be the one marked *A: How to make up for the harmful effects of living against gravity.* The reason is that, if a person had time for only one of the above-mentioned *Missing Link* portions, it is just possible that the techniques of counteracting the ill effects of gravity may *all by themselves* get some or most of the other jobs done. But that is a very "iffy" speculation. Even with the best application of one portion of the Missing Link, you are likely to regain health but not keep it. By employing all the above techniques you can rejuvenate and *maintain* your good health.

Index